YOUR
GENIUS
BODY

{ *A Guide for Optimizing Your Genes & Changing Your Life* }

ANDREW ROSTENBERG, DC

DISCLAIMER

The author does not assume any liability for the misuse of information in this book. The information is offered to provide you with beneficial concepts regarding your health and well-being. Please consult your primary care physician before beginning any nutrition or supplement program.

Every attempt has been made to provide accurate and effective information; the author and his book do not guarantee results.

Editing: Lisa Theobald (www.linkedin.com/in/lisa-theobald-2a879810/)
Graphic Design: Kendra Cagle (5LakesDesign.com)

Printed in the United States of America.
ISBN: 978-0-578393-26-1

Andrew Rostenberg
Red Mountain Natural Medicine
6434 W. Interchange Lane
Boise, ID 83709
208-322-7755

www.redmountainclinic.com
www.beyondmthfr.com

TABLE OF CONTENTS

HOW TO USE THIS BOOK

Dear Reader,

I wrote this book for both doctors and patients, in the hope that more people will learn about functional medicine and epigenetics by understanding how the science supports the natural way to health versus our drug-dependent healthcare model. For those in the medical profession who are interested in learning more about the ideas in this book, so that you can help your patients get better results, we offer a functional medicine coaching and practice management program called Beyond Genetics. As a chiropractor and functional medicine doctor myself, I had to figure out all these concepts and clinical protocols more or less from scratch. It took me years and thousands of hours of work to get to this point. I believe many others would benefit from this information, and that is why Your Genius Body was created.

If you want to dig in and start applying the ideas and concepts in this book, please reach out to us at Beyond Genetics. Send us an e-mail to support@ beyond-genetics.com, and we will send you information about our upcoming learning opportunities. You may also find information about our functional medicine coaching program on our Beyond Genetics website.

If you are a patient yourself or have a sick friend or loved one, please don't hesitate to contact our office at the e-mail above or call us directly at 208-322-7755. We would be honored to help you uncover the root cause of your health challenge and find natural ways to optimize your genes and change your life. We work with patients all over North America and from more than twenty different countries, and there is room for you too.

I hope you are as excited as I am about applying these new ideas to help more people!

Yours in Health,
Dr. Andrew Rostenberg

ACKNOWLEDGMENTS

There is not enough space here to thank all the individuals that have helped this book become a reality, but I will mention a few key individuals. I would like to thank Dr. Allen Roberds for introducing me to chiropractic and the healing power of innate intelligence, and for setting me on a path to becoming a healer myself. Dr. Robert Rakowski deserves credit for showing me the power of AK and functional medicine, and for inspiring me to investigate the all-important methylation cycle. Sterling Hill has been an inspiration for my own research, and without her work raising awareness of MTHFR and related problems, I would not be where I am today. Of course there are countless unknown PhD's and scientists who work throughout the world, investigating how our gut, genes, nutrition and environment influence our health - we would not be where we are today without all their efforts. And, finally, none of this would be possible without the love and support from my wife Mary and my three amazing children—Wes, Benji, and June.

PREFACE

I wrote this book because I believe we need to change our understanding of health and the potential of the human body. I am tired of watching a supposedly wealthy nation endure insane levels of cancer, heart disease, dementia, and diabetes. As a parent of young children, I am shocked at the rates of autism, depression, anxiety, ADD, ADHD, and sensory processing problems that were unheard of a generation ago. I am concerned about how many of my friends and neighbors are living with chronic inflammatory diseases such as Crohn's, ulcerative colitis, lupus, celiac disease, and more.

As I see more and more people diagnosed with cancer, I am beginning to wonder if our healthcare system knows only how to fight disease, not cure or prevent it. If we are so wealthy and smart, why are so many people so sick? Perhaps money is at the root of this issue, for as the old political axiom goes, "there is no money in solving problems, only in perpetuating them." It is ironic that despite all our access to science and information, we seem to be collectively less educated about our bodies today than ever before.

Many people do not realize that more than 30 million published peer-reviewed studies are catalogued in PubMed databases online. That enormous, mind-boggling amount of research represents the efforts of untold numbers of doctors and researchers spanning more than 100 years. Despite the fact that this information is full of references proving that natural medicine works, our healthcare system doesn't seem to pay much attention to it. The same cannot be said for those chiropractors, naturopaths, holistic MDs, and others who have been leading the alternative healthcare revolution for decades.

This book would not be possible without this rich source of online peer-reviewed data. I am indebted to the countless PhDs who have published thousands of papers proving how herbs, vitamins, plants, and food are the most effective tools for keeping us healthy. Many patients now recognize that in order to succeed with difficult and chronic cases, a doctor must read, study, and apply the very latest science. Luckily for them—and for you, dear reader—this book is full of exactly that kind of information. If you love to learn, this book will make you happy.

This book provides a roadmap for understanding what good health really means and how to create it naturally. You will learn how to solve many complex and chronic health problems naturally, to leverage your knowledge of the importance of genetics so that you can live a better life. Despite the many shortcomings and crises within healthcare, this book is not about bashing conventional medicine. We need drugs and surgeries, because in certain cases they save lives. But we don't need a medical system that uses dangerous and expensive drugs and surgeries to fix problems that can be easily and naturally treated.

Medicine is also crippled by the pharmaceutical industry, which is more interested in creating lifelong drug consumers than solving health problems. There just isn't money to be made from people who are healthy or dead, so the goal is get more people stuck in between. If our current health system was yielding satisfactory results, books like this wouldn't need to be written. But our health system is in crisis, and it is time for us to get educated about alternative healthcare that saves money and saves lives. Shouldn't the goal of our healthcare system be to reduce costs while improving our lives?

INTRODUCTION

We never know how far reaching something we may think, say, or
do today will affect the lives of millions tomorrow.

—B.J. Palmer

Before I get down into the nitty-gritty details of our genes and the biological systems of the human body, you need to remember the big picture—our genes are only as healthy as the environment in which they live. Americans are more chronically ill today than at any other time in history, and although we may want to blame our genes, they are not the root cause. The big reason why we are so sick is that we have created a toxic environment for our cells, our bodies, and our minds, and our genes are simply doing their best to cope with a bad situation. We must realize that the environment around us and within us is in constant communication with our genes. As you will soon see, when the environment is sick and unhealthy, so are we.

Throughout this book, I will help you connect dots between our genes, our health, and the environment inside our bodies. This book will shed light on the hidden connections and the root causes of why so many are so sick. We will travel on this path all the way from the digestive tract to the brain, and down into our genetic code and neurotransmitters. I will share with you clues, lessons, and insights that will forever change the way you look at human health.

One big idea in this book is the concept of epigenetics, which literally means "above the genes." Epigenetics is the study of how the environment inside our bodies turns our genes on and off. It explains how our DNA is activated by the choices we make, giving us the power to determine our fate regardless of the genes our parents gave us. Although the field of epigenetics and DNA research is fairly new, we don't have to wait fifty years before we can start applying this amazing science. As you will learn in the chapters that follow, we already have the necessary science and tools we need to fix most chronic health problems without drugs or surgery. It is no longer a matter of *if* we have the science; it is simply a matter of our willingness to apply what we already know.

Another major issue in this book is the methylation cycle, a biochemical pathway that influences and contributes to a wide range of crucial bodily functions, including immune function, detoxification, inflammation control, energy production, and more. Methylation problems make our bodily systems less flexible and less elastic in the face of health-negative environmental stimuli such as toxic heavy metals, chemical overloads, stressful and painful life experiences, and chronic infections. These problems make it harder for the body to right itself, to maintain balance and equilibrium, and to create health in the face of modern health challenges.

We are living in a toxic world full of bacteria, viruses, cancer-causing chemicals, psychological and emotional stresses, electromagnetic pollution, and more—that much we can all agree on. And while some people seem to be sensitive to the smallest amount of toxin exposure, others have a body that appears more robust and resilient. I, too, have noticed this discrepancy and have learned that the methylation cycle is largely responsible for the individual differences we see in our health. Genes make us all unique, and methylation is all about turning genes on (expressing) and off (repressing). It holds the genetic leverage to control who gets sick and who doesn't. No other system in our body impacts so much of who we are as the methylation cycle.

In sports, relationships, or health, the rule is always the same: it is impossible to come up with our next move if we cannot see our current position. You may be reading this book because of a sick child or family member who hasn't gotten better with traditional medicine approaches. Perhaps you have been sick yourself and have been unable to find an answer, despite going to 5, 10, or even 20 different doctors. Regardless of how you found this book, here you will find solutions that have proven enormously effective for thousands of patients. As you read, I believe you will agree that your body is amazing, and that working with, rather than against, the body is the best way to health. The goal of this book is to help you create health—abundant, radiant, natural health. To get there, we will take an honest, objective look at the human body and recognize that each of our bodies is, in fact, perfect. You have a genius body!

1.

_____

YOUR GENIUS BODY

The doctor of the future will give no medicine but will interest his patients in the care and maintenance of the human frame.

—Thomas Edison

I am more convinced than ever that the body is perfect. It never makes mistakes—not for the preterm infant fighting for her life, the elderly man with kidney failure, the woman battling breast cancer, or the teenager battling depression. Nowhere and never does the body err. It simply doesn't happen. The body always makes the right choice necessary to preserve and maintain life. No matter the insult, the injury, or the challenge, the body moves resources, turns on and off genes, and makes zero mistakes in its effort to keep us alive and healthy. No matter your health challenge, you always have a powerful force helping you—your own genius body.

Although the body is perfect and a genius, it is not invincible. It can be broken, drained, strained, stressed, and made very ill. Just ask my 47-year-old patient, Susan. Due to years of high stress at work and home, including a nasty divorce, a special needs child, and ongoing financial problems, her health crashed. A competitive athlete in college, she could now barely get off the couch. She suffered from years of pain, worry, anxiety, digestive upset, poor sleep, and very low energy. She tried to find answers by searching online and seeking help through the medical profession. Unfortunately, no answers came other than drugs to numb the pain and referrals for psychological evaluation. After going to literally dozens of doctors and spending a small fortune on tests, travel, and other expenses, she was close to her breaking point, emotionally and financially. Hope, it seemed, was all but lost when she first came to see me.

Susan was willing, despite her years of getting nowhere, to give another doctor one more chance. Like many patients, she came to my clinic with the attitude that "this was it," and I was her last hope. I wish I could say this is a rare occurrence, but in the world of chronic disease, patients like Susan are far too common. It was immediately clear that her biggest issue when she walked into my office that day was not her fatigue, her anxiety, or her digestive problems—her biggest issue was how she viewed her problems. She believed she would be sick forever, and I know that when we tell ourselves something over and over, we start to believe it, whether it's true or not. Susan needed help to see that her body wasn't completely broken.

Susan's healing started in the first five minutes, when I shared how her body never makes mistakes and how it is responding perfectly to the environment at all times. I helped her see her situation not as a curse from broken pathways and bad genes, but as an intelligent response by a genius body to an impossible situation. Although there was much more to do for her at this point, reframing her struggle helped her to see that her body could heal.

You can't hit a target that you can't see. And you can't heal if you convince yourself that your body is broken and defective. Truth is, despite the challenges your body faces, every second of every day, it makes the best decisions possible to produce the greatest positive outcomes, no matter what kind of health problem you have. The more you work with your body and help it do what it is trying to do, the better your results. That means fewer painkillers and antacids, less drugs and surgeries, and more health, happiness, and healing. I have experienced the miracles of what the body can do in my own life and practice; by the end of this book, you will be ready to experience them also.

By looking at our genes, we can gain an appreciation and understanding of why certain things have happened to us and to our loved ones. But we can go further than simply finding the genetic risks; we can change the environment we live in and thus change our genetic expression for the better.

OUR HEALTH IN DECLINE

Starting around the end of World War II, our bodies have been under constant assault from modern chemical and agricultural practices. Each generation has gotten progressively sicker with chronic disease. We have ignored the good from our past and embraced convenience and progress without thinking about the long-term costs. The "Illness Continuum" graph shown below helps to summarize the loss of health and increase in chronic disease during the last 60 to 70 years.

The Illness Continuum

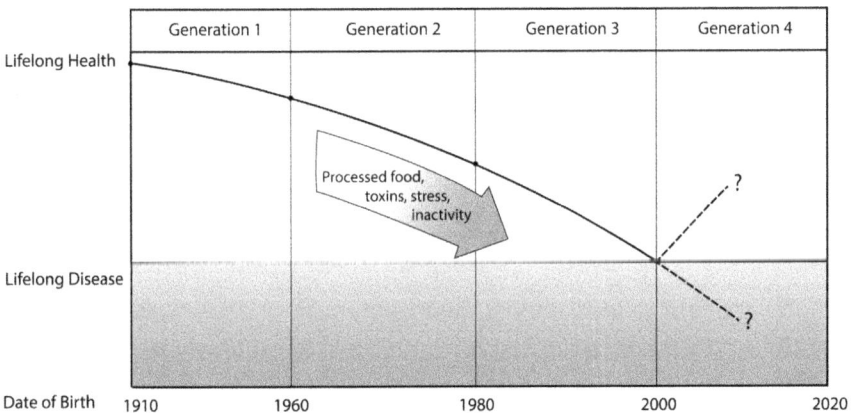

Figure 1.1 - *Each generation is now sicker than the one that preceded it. We can change our fate by optimizing our genes and environment, or we will suffer even more chronic disease.*

What is next for our society if this trend continues? Are we going to sit back and do nothing, or are we going to educate ourselves and rebuild a stronger foundation and home? Right now, it doesn't look good for our children's chances to be healthy. Unless we take charge and teach ourselves how to create health naturally by honoring our genetics and optimizing our lifestyles, our children will experience less health and well-being than their parents. This isn't just my opinion; researchers are also sounding the alarm.

For the past 10 years, Harvard researcher Dr. David S. Ludwig has been warning that the obesity epidemic will lead to a significant reduction in lifespan for children today compared to their parents. As a result of obesity, toxins, genetically altered foods, and physical inactivity, the current generation of children are living with diseases such as stroke, cancer, heart disease, and diabetes—childhood health issues that were unheard of just a few decades ago. This is the mother of all wake-up calls! The antidote to this problem is the same solution you will hear over and over in this book: To optimize our health, we must optimize our genes, and that means creating healthy environments and supporting the methylation cycle. I promise you if we all did enough of that, the world would change.

THE DOCTOR OF THE FUTURE

At a recent seminar, I heard a brilliant colleague of mine, Dr. John Bandy, a chiropractor and kinesiologist, say that "philosophy never changes, but the evidence always does." I thought this was a keen observation the moment I heard it. Science is constantly changing as our information and points of reference evolve. And if we base our philosophy on the ever-changing evidence, our philosophy is always changing. And a philosophy that constantly changes is really just an opinion. It is precisely the unchanging nature of philosophy that makes it useful and the changing nature of opinions that does the opposite. When everything around us is changing and wavering, our philosophy holds strong and guides our path. This doesn't mean we stop pursuing science, however. Instead, we maintain our philosophy that the body is perfect and intelligent, and that healing comes from within, while we look for the hard evidence to make our interventions more effective, natural, and safe.

If the doctor has no philosophy, no higher understanding of purpose or mission, he or she simply becomes a highly educated mechanic. Mechanics are great for cars, but that approach doesn't work for human health. The human body is not a machine; it is an organism housing life, energy, and consciousness that is capable of self-correction. The body will heal itself when the conditions change inside the body to create health. Remove what is offending the body and add what is needed, and the body will heal itself. A doctor simply must determine what needs to be removed–foods, chemicals, toxins, physical traumas, etc.–and design a program around a patient's individual needs. This is what the doctor of the future is all about.

The future of healthcare belongs to doctors who use nature and the human body's own innate healing potential as their main tools. In fact, if we approach healing and healthcare with an open mind, it is apparent that the body's own intelligence to right itself is superior to anything mankind can discover or invent.

When each of us is properly educated about the functions of our own body, each of us will in fact become our own doctor. In other words, the doctor of the future will be the educated patients themselves! By learning how to listen to the signals in our body, each of us will have the power to self-correct many of the common problems we all face. Although this idea will undoubtedly give pharmaceutical companies and hospital administrators heartburn, it is the only way out of our current predicament. In the future, doctors will teach their patients how to heal and give the power back to the patients. This is the revolution in healthcare that we desperately need.

2.

————

WHAT IS METHYLATION?

Everything should be made as simple as possible, but no simpler.

—Albert Einstein

Susan learned about methylation during countless hours of searching and reading online for ways to improve her health. Based on all she learned, she knew in her heart that methylation was a key factor to her health issues. Yet, like many patients, she didn't know what to do with the information. She had genetic testing and then used MTHFRSupport. com to produce a 50-plus-page variant report. She tried to figure out what the report meant and how the genes she had inherited had caused her body to crash during the high stress periods of her life. By the time she came to our office, she felt more confused than ever and even a little depressed about all she had read online.

As you research and learn more about methylation, you will see it is often referred to as the methylation cycle, which is depicted in Figure 2.1. For those of you who are new to the world of methylation, focus on the names of the chemicals presented here, because you will see these names repeated many times in the pages that follow. They will make more sense as we move along.

The methylation cycle occurs in every cell in our body, billions of times per second, from the moment of conception until our last breath. In the same way that computers work with 1s and 0s to produce instructions in binary code, our body uses methyl groups and the process of methylation to pass on information. For a visual of how this cycle works refer to Figure 2.1.

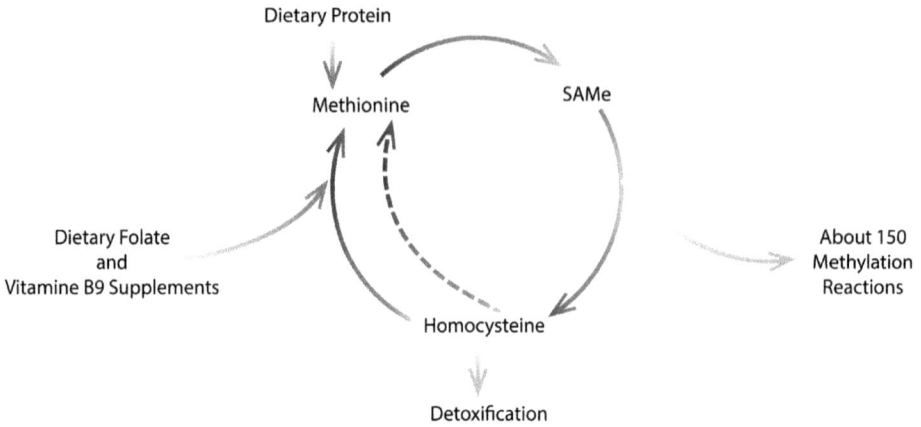

Figure 2.1 - *A simplified view of the methylation cycle*

The methylation cycle is responsible for the following:

- Maintaining DNA and RNA, the genetic material needed for cells to grow and divide

- Controlling methionine, an amino acid needed for protein synthesis

- Controlling neurotransmitters such as dopamine, adrenaline, and serotonin

- Controlling glutathione, the most important antioxidant in the body

- Controlling cysteine, an amino acid needed for detoxification and antioxidant production

- Controlling sulfate, the most important molecule for detoxification, growth, and repair

- Controlling metallothionein, a detoxifier of heavy metals such as lead and mercury

- Controlling taurine, which produces bile, increases GABA, prevents seizures, and protects the heart against arrhythmia

- Controlling SAMe, the main methyl donor and cofactor for all the body's methylation reactions

- Controlling homocysteine, a waste product related to stroke, heart disease, and dementia

When you look at all pathways involved, it is no wonder that doctors and patients alike have become obsessed with learning as much as they can about methylation. Any part of our chemistry that can influence so much of our health deserves a lot of attention. And as you work your way through this book, you will, like hundreds of my patients before you, find the answers to why optimizing your genes and your methylation cycle creates lasting, life-changing results.

AN OVERVIEW OF THE METHYLATION PROBLEM AND MTHFR

I like to describe the methylation cycle as an economy. Instead of dollars and liquid assets, we instead talk about methyl groups and vitamins. The names are different but the concepts are the same. When there are enough dollars in circulation, people are able to buy what they need and save for the future, bank accounts are full, and the pace of the economy is swift. When there aren't enough dollars or assets, people don't have money to spend, savings accounts are destroyed, and economic activity slows down.

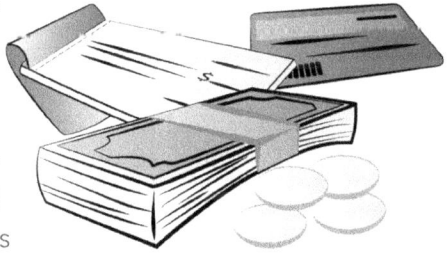

Now think of the same feast-or-famine scenario, but replace dollars and assets with methyl groups and vitamins. When the methylation cycle is working well and the diet and digestion are optimized, there are plenty of methyl groups available for the body to run all its complicated processes to keep us balanced and healthy. When the methylation cycle is slowed down, either by genetics, toxins, stress, or unhealthy food consumption (or a combination of all of those), there is a deficiency of methyl groups and related vitamins. With this deficiency comes pain, suffering, chronic disease, and a general inability to feel amazing, optimized, and healthy. Hold onto this metaphor and return to it as needed throughout the book to keep reminding yourself how simple this all can be.

The real Achilles' heel for people with methylation problems is that they cannot produce enough activated folate to meet the body's needs. Folate, Mother Nature's number one supplier of methyl groups, can impact the form of any growing tissue in the body. And to complicate the issue, our body's needs are always changing based on the demands of the environment. The environment might be sunny and warm one day, and stormy and cold the next. We might fall in love or receive a bonus for a job well done, or we might go without sleep for several nights with a sick child or suffer the grief of the unexpected loss of a loved one. To remain healthy, our bodies must be able to adapt to these changing conditions. That adaptation requires folate and methyl groups to perform the critical functions of epigenetics.

EPIGENETICS AND THE ENVIRONMENT

The reason that our lifestyle is more important than our genes has to do with an amazing process called epigenetics. Epigenetics describes how the environment controls our health by turning genes on and off. This gene regulation process occurs regularly every day in every cell in our body. Epigenetics controls how cells differentiate: cells with identical DNA differentiate to make a brain cell look and act differently from a heart cell, for example. Epigenetics also occurs when genes respond to environmental factors. No matter whether we inherited "good" genes or "bad" genes, the environment must trip the epigenetic switch for a health problem to manifest.

To get sick and stay sick for weeks, months, or years at a time, you must have a toxic, stressful environment that forces your body to turn on "bad" genes. This epigenetic response to a negative environment results in inflammation, toxicity, pain, depression, and low energy. To get healthy, you can increase healthy environmental signals with diet, exercise, nutrition, and lifestyle changes to allow your body to turn on "good" genes. It's just that simple! Fix the environment around your cells and you can change your life.

I consistently educate my patients that genes are only part of a bigger picture that includes our method of birth, childhood health issues, digestion, antibiotic exposure, sleep patterns, toxic chemicals and metals exposure, nutritional status, and structural traumas. Before I discuss specific genes with my patients, I always point out that the environment rules the roost. We must be crystal clear that genes respond to our environment in a dynamic fashion every day, all day. There is always an environmental component, some triggering event inside the body, that initiates the disease process. It would be detrimental if we focused only on genes, while ignoring lifestyle and environment—the true controllers of our destiny.

If you want proof that most genetic problems on their own don't cause disease, remember that people who have normal methylation genes contract diseases all the time. People without genetic methylation issues can get the same types of diseases—depression, cancer, heart disease, gallbladder disease, and chronic fatigue—that plague the methylation-impaired. Remember that every thought, action, and habit we have influences our health as much as or even more than our genes. To some, this may sound like heresy, but I am willing to bet that after reading this book you will agree. Yes, our genetics predispose us to certain limitations. But to say they are a curse is to avoid placing responsibility where it belongs—on how the environment has impacted our bodies over time. Believe me, a bad lifestyle is worse than a bad genetic report.

The big difference between people with methylation issues and the rest of the population is that people with methylation issues often get sicker quicker and stay sicker for longer periods of time. These folks are more sensitive to vaccines, toxins, pesticides, and other environmental stressors than individuals who don't possess these genetic imbalances. In fact, research indicates that 98 percent of autistic individuals have methylation problems, and that people with methylation issues have higher rates of cancer, heart disease, and depression.[1, 2, 3, 4] Methylation problems aren't the only factors involved in these diseases, but they absolutely raise your risk for contracting them. People with methylation problems must get the proper support their bodies need to prevent unnecessary pain, suffering, and dysfunction.

THE MTHFR PROBLEM

One particular enzyme produced in the methylation cycle, methylenetetrahydrofolate reductase (MTHFR), can have a huge impact on our lives. MTHFR looks like an abbreviation for something that would get a school boy in trouble for shouting on the playground. But don't let that fool you; it is a real issue causing real harm. The MTHFR gene has a serious impact on our health. MTHFR is by far the most important methylation gene and one that has received the most attention by researchers, scientists, doctors, and patients. I began my journey into the world of methylation by studying the MTHFR gene just like many of you. It makes a great starting point to provide an overview of what we are really facing when we talk about living with methylation imbalances.

MTHFR is generating a lot of interest, and for good reason. People who have been sick or have a sick loved one are searching for any genetic or biochemical issues that might be getting in the way of healing. When we study methylation, we realize that any problem in the cycle would have a powerful impact on health. Many biochemical pathways are affected by methylation, and *anything* that slows methylation can put our health at risk.

Inheriting Genes

−/− means neither one of your parents gave you a copy.

+/− means only one of your parents gave you a copy.

+/+ means both your parents gave you a copy.

Not everyone has problematic MTHFR genes, but those who do have a more challenging time producing enough methyl groups to meet all the body's needs. Under times of stress, toxic exposure, or poor digestion/poor nutrition, these individuals' bodies tend to run out of methyl donors faster and they get sick quicker. And in our modern world full of constant stress, high toxin loads, and poor food quality, people with MTHFR problems simply have higher rates of chronic disease.

Our lives depend not just on a steady supply of methyl groups, but on how well we use them inside our bodies. And this is where the MTHFR gene mutations come into play. I don't agree with the term "mutation," since nearly half the population has some form of this problem. I prefer the dry, scientific label, "single nucleotide polymorphisms," or SNPs for short. The word "polymorphism" means that a gene has several (poly) changes (morphism) to its normal or "wild type" code. Polymorphism means that the gene in question has been slightly changed by switching around the amino acids in the DNA at one or more locations.

Let's say, for example, a particular gene is made up of a thousand amino acids, and one of the amino acids gets changed. This doesn't destroy the gene, but it does change the gene's DNA slightly, potentially leading to a protein that isn't the exact right shape or isn't resistant to heat, so it breaks apart too fast. This is what happens with MTHFR and many, many other genes we investigate. The SNPs to the MTHFR gene change the shape and alter how well it stands up to heat, causing the protein to slow down and be destroyed by body heat. Regardless of whether we call it a mutation, imbalance, or SNP, the issue is real and does impact our health.

At the end of the day, the MTHFR SNPs of concern are known as the C677T, the A1298C, or a combination of both (called compound heterozygous). Science has named every SNP based on where it is located on the gene, and this is where the numbers come from. (Don't worry–they won't be on the midterm exam. Just recognize that different numbers represent different SNPs. All of this will make more sense once you have performed a genetic test and had your results properly interpreted. For information on how to do that, jump to the appendix, where I walk you through the process.)

> ## The Big 3 M T H F R SNP Problems
>
> ---
>
> *A1298C +/+: 30–40%
> loss of function*[5]
>
> *C677T +/+: 60–70%
> loss of function
> and sensitive to heat*[5]
>
> *Compound Hetero A1298C
> +/– and C677T +/–:
> 50–60% loss of function*

The actual numbers continue to be fine-tuned, but the research shows that 30 to 60 percent of the population has at least one copy, or variation, of a slowed MTHFR gene.[6, 7] Most of you reading this have this issue in some way. If you inherit one copy of the problem SNP from each parent, then you have a +/+ designation. If you inherit only one problematic copy of the gene from one parent, you have a +/- pattern. And if you didn't inherit the SNP from either parent, it's a simple -/-. For MTHFR, MAO, COMT, and many other genes, you want to see -/-, because that means you don't have the SNP. (I explain the COMT and MAO genes in more detail in chapters 11 and 12.) From there, inheriting a +/- is better than a +/+, because when you get the imbalanced copy from both parents, the enzyme is more severely impacted.

By now, your eyes are starting to glaze over and I might be losing you. So, in the interest of keeping you moving forward, let's turn our attention to a short discussion of the physical signs of methylation issues. Methylation problems aren't just something we find on a saliva test; the problem is usually right in front of us once we know where to look.

METHYLATION PROBLEMS ARE STARING US IN THE FACE

As you may know, we use saliva or blood tests to determine a person's genetic makeup. I use saliva DNA testing every week in my practice, and it is certainly one way to figure out whether a patient has a methylation problem, but these tests can be time-consuming and expensive. And not everyone has access to testing to determine whether they have a methylation problem. There are faster ways to detect a methylation problem.

One quick and simple way is to look at your family history. If you have a family history of cancer, heart disease, or stroke, you can be sure that there are methylation problems in your family. This is the simplest, quickest, and least expensive tool to help determine your genetic makeup, but not everyone knows their family health history. Luckily, there is another, easier way to identify a methylation problem—by looking at the shape and symmetry of your body itself. To help illustrate this point, I'll start with a quote from one of my favorite pieces of research:

Folate metabolism can influence the final form of any growing tissue due not only to its participation in nucleic acid synthesis, but also to its known function in regulating DNA and protein methylation.[8]

The methylation cycle can affect not only how you feel, but how you look. Folate can impact the form of any growing tissue in the body. In fact, the direct relationship between problems in our methylation cycle and changes to our outward appearance sparked my imagination as a first-year chiropractic student years ago. Because chiropractors are experts in structural alignment, I was fascinated that a vitamin had the potential to change the physical shape and structure of the human body. Once that seed was planted, I couldn't learn enough about the incredible methylation process. Along the way, I discovered many physical signs outside the body that point to a methylation problem on the inside.

The most important outward methylation sign I look for in patients is the epicanthal fold of the eye. This fold of tissue, which is shown in Figure 2.2, is basically an extra crease between the eye and the nose, and it is not present on everyone's face. Because this facial feature is so common in the Asian population, further research is needed to determine whether it indicates the presence of MTHFR or similar genes. However, in non-Asians, the epicanthal fold appears to be present *only in individuals who have a methylation issue.*

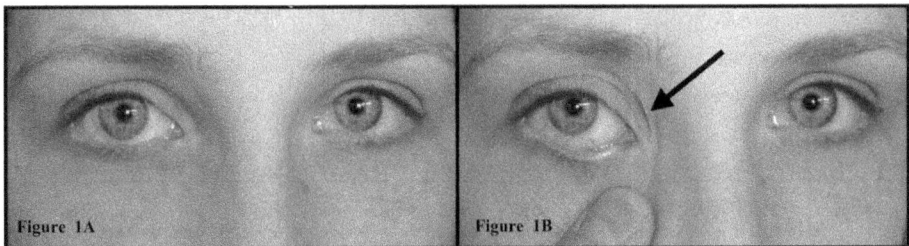

Figure 1A   Figure 1B

Figure 2.2 - *Some epicanthal folds will be easily visible; others will be "hidden" and can be seen only by pulling the skin downward (Figure 1B).*

Based on this idea, the presence of this sign indicates an individual has MTHFR-related issues. However, even if you don't have this outward sign, you can still have MTHFR and methylation imbalances, so don't take this as your only method of assessing MTHFR. It's just a quick tool and one that is, in my opinion, accurate in the high 90 percent range. I was shown this marker by a chiropractor and functional medicine doctor in Minnesota, Dr. Jeff Brist. Once he showed me this phenomenon, I started to notice it everywhere—on my friends, my family, and of course my patients.

Even though it is the easiest indicator to see, the epicanthal fold is not the only indicator you need to know about. Dozens of methylation markers will show up on the outside or inside of the body. Learning these patterns can help you quickly identify individuals who are in need of extra methylation support. The following chart (Figure 2.3) shows which physical characteristics and health problems suggest a methylation problem is involved.

Gestation	Childhood/Puberty	Adult Degeneration
Chromosal Nondisjunction	**Structural Findings**	**Chronic, Metabolic Disease**
• Down's • Turner's • Kleinfelter's • Fragile X • X X Y • X Y Y	• Pectus Excavatum • Arachnodactily • Epicanthal Folds • Limb Length Inequalities • Segmental and Hemivertebra • Scoliosis • Spina Bifida Oculta • Posterior Ponticles • Hypertelorism • Hypotelorism • Fetal Alcohol Syndrome	• Alzheimers • Stroke • Thrombosis • Embolism • Heart Disease • Peripheral Vascular Disease • Diabetes • Cancers • Myocardial Infarction • Environmental Illness • Infertility • Depression
Midline Congenital Defects		
• Cleft Palate • Arnold-Chiari • Malformation • Heart Defects • Horseshoe Kidney • Spina Bifida • Any Malformed Organ	**Neurological Findings** • Autism • Depression • Epilepsy • ADD/ADHD • Schizophrenia	

Figure 2.3 - *Methylation issues at different life and developmental stages*

Look at that list! Many of you probably see these patterns and conditions in your own family, your friends, and your co-workers. These physical characteristics are so common, in fact, that we don't realize they actually speak to a deeper issue of genetic methylation imbalance. It is safe to say that everyone reading this knows individuals with these unique physical signs.

There is strong evidence that connects methylation issues with changes in the physical symmetry of the body. Issues such as scoliosis and limb-length inequality aren't fully understood, but I believe they are probably manifestations of methylation problems. Although emerging research connecting folate to tissue shape is very exciting, we need more dedicated research to shed light on this phenomenon.

CONCLUSION

Our bodies perform miracles every day by moving, removing, shifting, trading, and recycling methyl groups from one molecule to the next. Methylation impacts everything from our genes to our gut and our brain. It impacts how we feel when we wake up and start our day, and it determines whether we age with health or with chronic disease. Optimum methylation is possible only when we have an abundant supply of methyl groups. A large percentage of people are born with MTHFR SNPs that affect how fast their methylation cycle can operate.

You've seen how important methylation is and how disruptions in methylation are related to serious metabolic and neurologic disease processes. But before you start blaming your health problems on your genes, remember that the environment controls your health through the process of epigenetics.

Recognizing a problem is the first step to fixing it. Hopefully by now you can see that methylation is a huge deal, a common problem, and something we all need to support—and that is what this book is all about. Before we venture into fixing specific health issues such as poor digestion, oxalate toxicity, anxiety, and more, we must spend a little more time on the basic biochemistry that underpins all this amazing science. After all, if you want to enjoy all the benefits of living with an optimized methylation cycle, you need to learn the fundamentals. With a solid understanding of the concepts behind MTHFR-related problems, you will reap the rewards. You will experience better health and become a source of inspiration and guidance for those around you who still suffer. The doctor of the future!

REFERENCES

1. Marvin, B., A. Goldblatt, J. Galanko, S. Jill James. Association of MTHFR gene variants with autism. *J Am Phys Surg* (2004) 9(4): 106-8.

2. Hsiung, Ting D., C. Marsit, et al. Global DNA methylation level in whole blood as a biomarker in head and neck squamous cell carcinoma. *Cancer Epidemiology Biomarkers & Prevention* (2007) 16(1): 108-14.

3. Banecka-Majkutewicz, Z., W. Sawula, et al. Homocysteine, heat shock proteins, genistein and vitamins in ischemic stroke–pathogenic and therapeutic implications. *Acta Biochim Pol* (2012) 59(4): 495-99.

4. Wei, J., J. Xu, X. Lu, et al. Association between MTHFR C677T polymorphism and depression: a meta-analysis in the Chinese population. *Psychology, Health & Medicine* (2016) 21(6): 675-85.

5. Gokcen, C., N. Kocak, A. Pekgor. Methylenetetrahydrofolate reductase gene polymorphisms in children with attention deficit hyperactivity disorder. *Int J Med Sci* (2011) 8(7): 523-28.

6. Wilcken, B., F. Bamforth, S. Li, et al. Geographical and ethnic variation of the 677C> T allele of 5, 10 methylenetetrahydrofolate reductase (MTHFR): findings from over 7000 newborns from 16 areas world wide. *Journal of Medical Genetics.* (2003) 40(8): 619-25.

7. Leclerc, D., S. Sibani, R. Rozen. Molecular Biology of Methylenetetrahydrofolate Reductase (MTHFR) and Overview of Mutations/Polymorphisms. *Madam Curie Biosciences Database [Internet].* Austin, Texas: Landes Bioscience, 2000-2013. www.ncbi.nlm.nih.gov/books/NBK6561/. Accessed December 26, 2016.

8. Aneiros-Guerrero, A., A.M. Lendinez, A.R. Palomares, et al. Genetic polymorphisms in folate pathway enzymes, DRD4 and GSTM1 are related to temporomandibular disorder. *BMC Medical Genetics.* (2011) 12(1): 75-84.

3.

———

METHYLATION AND GENETICS

Your genes are not your destiny, but they are your tendency,
especially when you are under stress.

—Dr. R

Now that I have laid the groundwork of what methylation is and why it is so important, you should get familiar with a few more concepts before we move on to discussing how to fix methylation-related health problems. There is no easy way or shortcut to talk about genes and epigenetics without using words and ideas you likely haven't seen before. As you read this chapter, keep an open mind. When you encounter new words and ideas, just keep reading; it will make sense even if you don't have a PhD in biochemistry. In the chapters that follow, you'll learn more about how this all fits together. For now, consider this a crash course in epigenetics and health. I will do my best to keep it simple.

Not only does the body never make mistakes, but it is more complex than we will ever know. I'm a doctor and I am 100 percent comfortable with that idea; as a patient, you should be too. We don't need to know about every single miniscule physiological process inside our body to be healthy. A Zen monk once said, "When you are hungry, eat, and when you are tired, sleep, for this is the secret to happiness." Do not overcomplicate the road to health. I see many chronic patients who have researched so much on their own that they are confused: They have no idea what to eat, are unsure how to supplement their diet, and are completely lost in the minutia. That is called "analysis/paralysis," and it can happen to any of us. It's okay to be lost as long as you are wise enough to stop and ask for directions.

So don't give up if you feel a little lost so far. I promise things will get simpler as we move along. I often tell my patients that if you are willing to be confused, you will learn a lot! The difference between those who learn a great deal and those who do not is simple: Many people stop and give up when they get confused; others take it as a challenge and work harder to solve the problem, learn, and grow. I'm in the latter category and I hope that you are too. With so many problems that need solving, we need to learn everything we can.

> *Susan's impression was that she was sick because of methylation, and she thought that a person's genetic makeup could never be changed. She didn't realize that genes are controlled by the environment, that the microbes in our gut include 100 times more genetic material than we have in our entire body, and that we are not victims of the genes we inherit. Just as I told her that the body never makes mistakes, I also explained how we create health despite the genes we inherit by optimizing our internal environment. We discussed how each gene that seemed to make something negative happen also provides a benefit in other situations. After hearing this, she let out a deep breath, relaxed her shoulders, and leaned forward, eager to hear more. The ah-ha! moment had arrived and she finally had a glimmer of hope that her health could improve. She was finally ready to start getting better.*

Methylation is a complicated word, but the definition is pretty simple. Methylation is a group of chemical reactions that involve four atoms: one carbon atom attached to three hydrogen atoms. Our entire complicated relationship of genetics, health, and disease literally comes down to a molecule made of these four atoms. These methyl groups must come from outside the body in the food we eat, and they are produced by bacteria in our gut. The human body does not create these molecules from scratch, so we need to consume a steady supply of nutrients to prevent dangerous deficiencies. Methyl groups are so important that without them, we can experience very serious health problems.

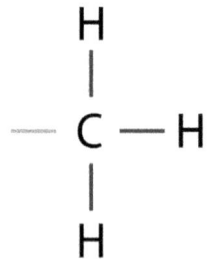

$$H$$
$$|$$
$$-\;C - H$$
$$|$$
$$H$$

Methyl group

3. Methylation and Genetics

In an ideal world, we would get all the methyl groups we need from an organic, unprocessed, high vegetable diet. We humans need to eat as many organic vegetables as we can. I am not implying that everyone should be a vegan or vegetarian to get enough methyl groups in their body; we also need animal protein such as fish, meat, and eggs, because they provide a substantial source of the B12 that is critical for many biochemical pathways, including methylation. Diets high in dairy, meat, wheat, corn, soy, and sugar are devoid of key vitamins and antioxidants and cause high levels of inflammation—a dangerous combination! The methyl groups we need come mainly from green plants such as spinach, lettuce, kale, asparagus, chard, and broccoli, as well as from beans and lentils. (Interestingly, the word foliage, which comes from the Latin word for leaf, is where the word folate, aka vitamin B9, comes from. Plant foliage is full of methyl groups, and so is vitamin B9.) If increasing vegetables is too hard to stomach, you can take supplements (such as B vitamins, choline, inositol, and folate) to bolster your supply of methyl vitamins. Researchers have developed supplements specifically for methylation issues, and you will read about many of them in this book.

Unfortunately, too many people continue to eat a diet of processed food, refined sugars, GMO toxins, fast foods, and the like. This type of convenience food is devoid of life-sustaining vitamins and leads to malnutrition and chronic disease. Living in a stressful, toxic world without a healthy methylation cycle is a recipe for disease and disaster.

Supplements High in Methyl Groups

_____

Methylfolate. MethylB12. Trimethylglycine. Methionine. Choline, and Betaine

A deficiency of methyl groups in our bodies can lead to cancer, heart disease, stroke, and depression through several different mechanisms.[1, 2, 3, 4] Additionally, research now shows that methylation is critical for preventing dementia, Alzheimer's disease, and Parkinson's disease, highlighting how methylation is key for healthy brain function as we age.[5, 6, 7]

Perhaps the biggest issue with methylation, however, is the effect it has on the unborn. If an adult has a problem with methylation, it may not impact too many of her cells, because many of her cells are fully grown and not dividing very quickly. But if she is pregnant and her baby runs out of methyl groups while in the womb, the child's rapidly growing cells could potentially have a deficiency of methyl groups. This is why women and men who want to start a family should be working to optimize their methylation *before* they get pregnant!

A QUICK LOOK AT GENETIC POTENTIAL

The body attaches or removes a methyl group on top of a gene to control whether a gene is expressed (turned on), or repressed (turned off). This gene regulation occurs regularly in normal development to make a brain cell look and act differently from a heart cell, for example. It also occurs when genes respond to environmental factors.

When a gene has a methyl group stuck to it, it is "methylated" and the gene is repressed. When a gene lacks a methyl group, it is "unmethylated" and the gene is expressed. If the environment is stressful, methyl groups are placed in a certain pattern, encoding the environmental stress directly into our genomes. Conversely, if the environment is calm and healthy, methyl groups are placed in a different pattern, reflecting the healthy environment. In this way, cells can store epigenetic information using methyl groups in a similar way to how your computer stores memory on its hard drive.

Regardless of the genes we were born with, our body's cellular environment controls which genes are expressed and which are repressed. As discussed in chapter 2, the environment signals to the cell and the cell makes changes to adapt to the environment. It is an elegant back-and-forth, a smart give-and-take that keeps our biology in balance. In fact, stem-cell biologist Bruce Lipton, PhD, stumbled upon this process way back in the 1960s. Dr. Lipton wrote about his powerful discoveries in his book *The Biology of Belief*, which offers evidence of how the environment truly controls the fate of the cell—and by extension the whole body![8]

Here is a mind-blowing thought to consider: According to the Human Genome Project, we humans have around 30,000 genes.[9] Each gene is either expressed or repressed; there is no being half-on or half-off. Given this reality, we use the equation of 2 to the 30,000th power ($2^{30,000}$) to represent all the possible combinations in our genome. Even though $2^{30,000}$ is a really big number, it still doesn't come close to our full potential. To find the true answer of our genetic potential, we will turn again to the wisdom of Dr. Lipton, who discovered that each gene can produce 30,000 different variations of a single protein. This means our math problem must change: Instead of $2^{30,000}$, we now have $30,000^{30,000}$ possible combinations in our genome. I am no mathematician, but I can assure you that $30,000^{30,000}$ is as close to infinity as our minds can understand.

Now take that amazing, mind-blowing idea and consider again how important the methylation cycle is to this process. Every cell and every piece of DNA depends on methyl groups to function properly. Our body's ability to express genes is 100 percent dependent on the methylation cycle. It seems that we have an infinite capacity for adapting, growing, and healing!

Figure 3.1 shows the methylation cycle again, but this time the genes and enzymes are shown. Look at where the MTHFR enzyme sits to see how a problem in that pathway will impact the rest of the cycle. This is why methylation problems can be so problematic, and why fixing them can be so profound.

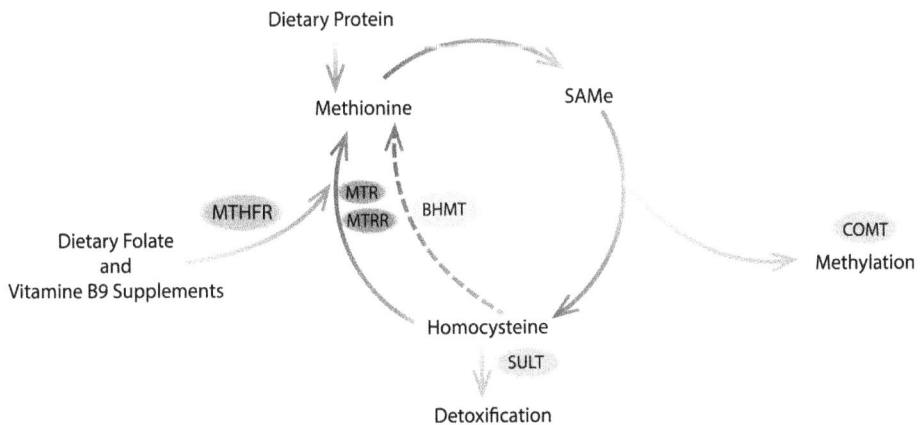

Figure 3.1 - *Simplified methylation cycle with major enzymes shown*

To get the bird's eye view of how methylation and genetics can change your life, you need to understand three new terms: genotypes, pheno-types, and haplotypes. Although it might not seem obvious now, learning the meanings of these terms will help you solve your frustrating, chron-ic, painful, and expensive health problems naturally. And isn't that what you're looking for?

GENOTYPE AND DNA

Your genotype includes the 20,000+ genes that create your unique, individual DNA–the genetic, unique you. It includes all your SNPs and all the genes you inherited from your parents–half from your mother and half from your father. Your genotype is the entire "deck of cards" that you are born with. It will always be the same and will never change. The genes you received at conception determine the color of your hair and eyes, and your skin pigment, sex, and other qualities about you that will never change. No one on Earth has the same genotype as you, unless you have an identical twin. Twins aside, every person on Earth has a unique genotype–7 billion genotypes and counting!

Your genotype is your unique DNA fingerprint, and it contains all the methylation-related genes you will hear about in the rest of the book: MTHFR, COMT, MAO, etc. Haven't heard of those genes before? Not to worry, because by the end of the book you will be well acquaint-ed! Throughout the book, you will learn which part of your genotype is most import-ant for health and healing. Fortunately, it is just a tiny fraction of the thousands of genes in your body. You'll need to understand only a few super-critical genes to start optimizing and changing your life.

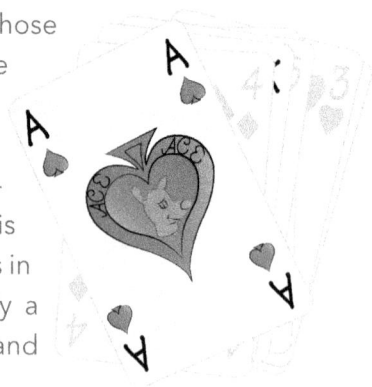

Will the "problem" genes you inherit express themselves and cause health issues? The answer to this is no, as long as you work to optimize the environ-ment and the epigenetics that control the genes. You can create health and optimum genetic expression simply by creating an optimal environment.

Genotyping has its own language and is confusing to anyone who is brave enough to sort through the research. You don't need me to tell you that this subject is complicated. However, you don't need to go very deep into the science to pull out the pearls you need. Your genotype, while extremely complex, can be listed in a simple format made available from companies that provide genetic testing. (For more information about genetic testing companies, see the appendix.)

PHENOTYPE

I tell my patients that another goal is to identify your phenotype, because once that is known, they can start to move forward. Be aware, however, that simply looking at a list of genes in isolation takes them out of context. Looking only at your genotype, while ignoring your phenotype and haplotype (discussed a bit later), is not a useful approach to treatment. It's impossible to prescribe vitamins and fix health problems effectively using only genotype information. Doing so will result in frustration, added expense, and lack of results that wastes time and energy. To treat methylation issues successfully, you must also look at your phenotype and the haplotype before deciding on a path to healing.

The phenotype is one of the most important parts of the methylation puzzle. It is the set of observable characteristics of an individual that result from the interaction of its genotype with the environment. In other words, if the genotype is the deck of cards, then the phenotype is how well your body can play the card game on your behalf. A phenotype is an *expression* of the genes, not the genes themselves.

Medicine uses named "diseases" to label patient characteristics—using terms such as obesity, depression, anxiety, cancer, irritable bowel, diabetes, etc. When doctors give a diagnosis of diabetes, diverticulitis, or depression, they aren't talking just about symptoms, but also about genes, pathways, and nutritional imbalances, even if they aren't aware of it. Every disease and symptom we experience is caused by environmental triggers that change how our genes are expressed. This is what the phenotype is all about. *There are as many phenotypes out there as there are types of chronic disease.* Luckily, each person usually has to battle just one or two dominant phenotypes at a time.

Because our phenotype is determined by how our genes interact with the environment inside and outside our body, the more stressful our environment, the stronger our phenotype becomes. The phenotype determines our body's tendency to experience a set of symptoms, or to develop a certain health problem, when it is under stress. For example, some people gain weight and use food to self-medicate when they are under chronic stress. Some people lose weight and start smoking to deal with excess emotional strain. Still others might experience insomnia, while some might have bloating, pain, and irritable bowel when feeling stressed out. Different people, different genes, different phenotypes. Everyone has a phenotype, a genetic tendency, that determines how their body will react when it is challenged. We cannot be overweight and underweight at the same time, or have high blood pressure and low blood pressure at the same time—we all have specific genetic tendencies that influence how our bodies react to stresses.

When we deal with our methylation disorders, our phenotype is why we feel sick or have symptoms in the first place. It's the reason we go to the ER or to the doctor's office. Our phenotype determines how our genetic SNPs plus environmental signals cause us to feel and function. For example, we cannot consciously feel our MTHFR gene, but we can feel depressed from the expression of the MTHFR gene, and depression is a well-known phenotype. Similarly, we can't feel our ACE, AGT, ADD1, or BMHT genes (which you'll learn about later), but we can have gallstones and chronic acid reflux, which are common phenotypes related to those genes. Depression, gallstones, and acid reflux are not simply genetic problems—they are phenotypes caused by the interaction of our genes and the environment over time.

Knowing your phenotype can help you predict how your methylation-related genes will react to stress, and the phenotype indicates what needs to be done to help treat the root cause of the problem. If you change the environment around your cells, the genes themselves will change their expression, and the phenotype will be improved.

For a better understanding of this concept, let's look at fatty liver disease, shown in figure 3.2, a preventable disease that is becoming more common in our society.

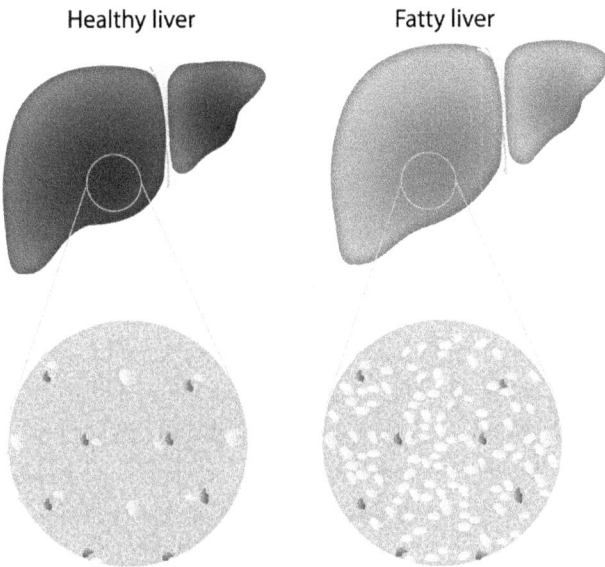

Healthy liver   **Fatty liver**

Figure 3.2 - *Fat tissue accumulates inside the liver, which creates inflammation, slowing down the liver's metabolic pathways.*

Fatty liver disease is estimated to affect one out of every three Americans—a whopping 100 million people.[10] We can be certain that not all people who have fatty liver are related. In other words, fatty liver disease affects millions of people who have millions of different genotypes. So if we cannot blame this disease on their genes, it must be the environment inside the body, and specifically the liver, that is the problem.

Similar to other complex, chronic diseases, fatty liver represents a unique phenotype—a collision between toxic environmental signals and the body's cellular response to the insult. Fatty liver disease is most often caused by changes in the liver's environment due to excess alcohol consumption, high-carbohydrate diets, poor digestion, and general nutritional deficiencies.

Enter methylation pathways, which affect not only how our cells grow and repair, but which also protect sensitive organs such as the liver from damage caused by toxins, stress, and inflammation. Because methylation vitamins—aka methyl donors—interact with our genetic code, they become critical factors in keeping our body and liver healthy. Methylation nutrients such as choline, betaine, B9, B12, and trimethylglycine (TMG) provide the chemistry necessary for the liver to function at its best.

Methyl donors are so important for the liver that they can actually prevent fatty liver disease. Normally when we (or other mammals) eat a diet high in refined carbohydrates and starches, the liver is full of triglycerides and becomes inflamed. Processing all those carbohydrates depletes the liver of key methylation vitamins such as B12, folate, choline, and betaine, and other fat-burning vitamins such as carnitine.[11] From a study published in 2009, we know that when rats are fed methyl donors such as betaine, they do not develop a fatty liver, even when placed on a high-fat diet.[12] Another study published in 2012 highlights the fact that when our bodies run out of methylation nutrients (methyl donors), we develop fatty livers and become predisposed to other problems such as metabolic syndrome, the risk factors associated with heart disease.[13]

Abusing alcohol, over-consuming carbohydrates, and suffering with poor digestion in general can cause the body to burn up its vitamin stores faster than they can be replaced. If this happens for a few days, the liver will be fine. But if it happens for weeks, months, or years, the body becomes progressively weakened and fatigued, and fatty liver is often a result.

Fatty liver disease is a perfect example of a phenotype. We know it's not caused by the genes; it's caused by an altered environment that has dangerously depleted the body of methyl donor nutrients—nutrients so powerful that they can prevent the progression of fatty liver once it has started.[14]

If changing our environment to increase our body's methyl donors can prevent and reverse damage caused by fatty liver, just imagine all the other health problems that can be prevented with methylation support.

The key here is to realize that fatty liver and other diseases can develop inside our body whether we have "good" or "bad" genes. It's not the genes that are at fault; it's the environment! And every serious health problem has a genetic component that can be improved by altering the environment within and around the cells themselves. This is what treating methylation problems is all about. As you will see repeatedly in the pages to follow, no group of nutrients is more important for a healthy cellular environment than the methyl donors.

The beautiful thing is that phenotypes (and diseases) can change when we treat the underlying cause of the condition (the environment). When we change the environment outside our body, we change the environment inside our cells, and we change the cells' genetic response. When we change the genetic response, we change our phenotype. When we begin to work on our methylation problem, we are beginning a journey that starts to unlock our true genetic potential.

In summary, the phenotype represents all our SNPs plus all of the environmental challenges—stresses, toxins, malnutrition, etc. When you add everything to solve the methylation puzzle, you need to pay attention to your phenotype. Trying to treat methylation issues without recognizing a phenotype will lead to lackluster results. Your phenotype helps you know where you need to start and helps you determine whether you are high in adrenaline or low, whether you are prediabetic or suffering with hypoglycemia, or whether you must heal the gut first or start supporting neurotransmitters with amino acids and methylation support.

PHENOTYPE VS. HAPLOTYPE: WHERE THE RUBBER HITS THE ROAD

Confused yet? Remember what I said earlier—your willingness to wade through this chapter, a little bit confused and a little bit curious, is necessary to increase your understanding. It might be a little painful right now, but stay with it, because I have a few more points to cover before we jump into the good stuff.

Although the genotype refers to all of the genes you inherited, and the phenotype refers to how we label your symptoms, the haplotype refers to your genes as a group.[15] In other words, your haplotype is a small group of really important genes that have an outsized impact on how your body works. It is interesting to point out that other people may have the exact same haplotype as you because they inherited the same set of methylation SNPs, even though you both have your own unique genotype.

To clarify this idea, let's look at a couple of examples. Upon testing their genotype, many people discover they have homozygous (two bad copies) of each gene MTHFR C677T +/+, COMT +/+, and MAO-A +/+. I see this pattern all the time. Everyone with this combination is said to share the same haplotype for those genes. I refer to this haplotype as the "high adrenaline, high anxiety, slow methylation haplotype." That is just my way of describing the pattern, because those are the most common symptoms I see in individuals with those genes. Common phenotypes in this group of individuals include anxiety, estrogen dominance, and adrenal fatigue.

Another example of a common problematic haplotype is someone who inherited bad copies of each of the following genes: GAD1, ACE, AGT, ADD1, COMT, MAO, and MTHFR A1298C. I call this haplotype "the high stress, neuroinflammation, low gut function, slow methylation haplotype." The phenotypes associated with this haplotype combo would be chronic fatigue, chronic GERD, irritable bowel, and fibromyalgia. Again, we're not looking at one gene, but multiple genes at once.

Let's briefly examine the genes and pathways involved in this second example. ACE, AGT, and ADD1 influence levels of angiotensin, a stress hormone made by our kidneys. When these SNPs are present, the body has elevated levels of angiotensin, and this reduces blood flow to the GI tract. Some studies show that these SNPs may even cause damage to the heart valve, since increases in blood pressure and cortisol usually accompany the increase in angiotensin.

GAD1 involves the breakdown of glutamate into GABA, a neurotransmitter that sends chemical messages through the brain and the nervous system and is involved in regulating communication between brain cells; the more GAD SNPs are present, the less efficient the body is at making GABA. This can lead to brain inflammation, since too much glutamate in the brain (glutamate, found in MSG, can be a toxin) leads to excess brain activity, seizures, and inflammation. With GAD1, the tendency is toward glutamate and away from GABA, which often leads to neurological symptoms that change behavior, mood, appetite, and more.

In addition, when you also have the COMT and MAO SNPs, your body will struggle to break down stress hormones such as adrenaline and norepinephrine. Individuals with COMT and MAO SNPs are usually highly intelligent, driven, and susceptible to burn-out and OCD issues.

Combine all of these genes into a functional haplotype—ACE, AGT, ADD1, GAD, COMT, MAO, and MTHFR A1298C—and you start to realize that each gene is influenced by other genes.

If you are treating a methylation problem, and you look only at your genotype but ignore your haplotype, you are going to have less than satisfactory results. Yet even looking at both the genotype and the haplotype will leave you falling short. To see the big picture and take good care of your body and treat methylation issues, you should study your genotype, appreciate your haplotype, and make sure you understand your phenotype!

SNPS CHANGE ENZYME SPEED

There is one more simple but important concept you need to understand before we move on to the next chapter: What does it really mean when we talk about genetic SNPs, or polymorphisms? This isn't a concept you see on the nightly news or hear about on NPR, so a little clarification won't hurt.

Single nucleotide polymorphisms, or SNPs, are not just mutations or a change in the genetic code. SNPs create changes in the speed of enzymes and alter the final shape and function of whatever protein or enzyme was supposed to be produced. When a gene has an SNP, it may end up being built a little bit differently, and depending on its shape, the SNP may either slow down the enzyme or speed it up. The real problem with SNPs such as MTHFR, COMT, MAO, SULT, and so on, is that when they change the speed of an enzyme, it can create a big impact on the body's chemistry. Growth, repair, and detoxification are all impacted by enzymes moving faster or slower.

When environmental signals (inflammation, stress, toxins, etc.) influence the cell to make more of an enzyme to meet local demands, the cell responds intelligently to select the best response to the stimuli. These signals are epigenetic, or above the gene, and they eventually cause DNA and then RNA to replicate. Increases in RNA cause the cell to increase production of specific proteins and enzymes.

Many of these proteins, such as MTHFR, MAO, COMT, GAD, and so on, are critical systems, and if slowed down will cause symptoms and phenotypes to occur. MTHFR and all the other methylation-related genes are just enzymes after all. Your DNA is the blueprint; the enzyme is the final product. When we consider methylation genetics as a cause of a health problem, we are also talking about enzymes causing the health problem.

It is impossible to understand methylation problems without realizing that a big part of the problem is the change in the speed of an enzyme. Methylation controls so many aspects of our biochemistry that anything that affects it will have profound effects across multiple bodily systems. Once enzymes are slowed down, however, we become less able to deal with changes in our environment without experiencing symptoms. When we cannot effectively adapt to changes in our environment, we develop chronic diseases that lower the quality and quantity of our lives.

Susan made amazing progress over the several months we worked together. By working on her gut-methylation-brain issues using the research included in this book, she was able to regain a healthy life. It didn't happen by chance, and it didn't happen overnight, but over the course of three months, Susan finally reached her destination in three important steps.

Her first step was to recognize that her body doesn't make mistakes. The body simply does everything it can every second of your life to keep you healthy and balanced. Susan made some room in her mind for the possibility that her body wasn't broken and that it had the capacity to heal. That opened the door for the next big thing to happen.

The second step for her was acknowledging that the environment controls the genes. By taking ownership of the environment surrounding her body, she started to improve how her genes functioned. Susan agreed that to give her body a chance to heal, she needed to improve her sleep hygiene, change her diet, and reduce unnecessary stress. She also acknowledged that in order to see the big picture, she would need to do some testing and also use supplements to augment her diet and digestion.

Susan's third step was all about taking action. She performed in-depth functional medicine testing through our office, which included blood work, genetic testing via saliva, and urine organic acid testing. We carefully analyzed her results and discovered her biochemical weaknesses that included Candida overgrowth, oxalate toxicity, and methylation imbalances. She also inherited homozygous (two bad copies) of the MTHFR C677T, COMT, and MAO genes—a triple whammy of genetic SNPs.

She was eager to attack everything we found, but I had to remind her that we had to start with the gut before addressing the brain, mitochondria, and methylation cycle. We started with supporting her gut and helping get her oxalate problem under control. After a couple weeks, she was noticing better sleep and almost no pain, and her energy was starting to increase. Over the next few months, we moved away from gut-based support and began to help lower her excess levels of catecholamines, replenish her B-vitamin stores, and optimize her methylation cycle *with activated forms of folate and B12. By the 90-day mark, she was 20 pounds lighter and off her medications with zero pain, and she rode her bicycle for 45 minutes for the first time in years. She had optimized her genes and changed her life. You can do the same by reading and applying the pearls I am sharing with you in the rest of this book.*

CONCLUSION

You have learned a lot in this chapter. Recognizing that genetics is a seriously complicated issue, you've moved beyond confusion to learn some key ideas that will help you put everything into context. You now know that the genotype is your own unique DNA fingerprint. You know that phenotypes result when your genes are influenced by your environment over time. You might end up with a diagnosis and a set of symptoms, but those are still just different types of phenotypes. And you now recognize the idea of a haplotype—different combinations of individual genes.

Even if you stop reading here, you know more about methylation than most doctors do! You can apply these ideas right now and start healing your methylation cycle and turn your life around for the better. But if you are like me and prefer to experience the absolute most abundant health possible, continue reading, because the good stuff is yet to come!

Despite any inborn limitations with regard to enzyme speed, if you deal with issues of MTHFR and beyond, you can still be radiantly healthy, despite your genes. To achieve this, you can start at 30,000 feet and look at your health and your life from a distance, before you dive into the molecular and atomic world. You need a correct big picture before you zoom in and start getting finicky with the details. Got it?

REFERENCES

1. Li, P., C. Qin. Methylenetetrahydrofolate reductase (MTHFR) gene polymorphisms and susceptibility to ischemic stroke: a meta-analysis. *Gene.* (2014) 535(2): 359-64.

2. Kolb, A.F., L. Petrie. Folate deficiency enhances the inflammatory response of macrophages. *Mol Immunol.* (2013) 54(2): 164-72. PMID: 23280395

3. Słopien, R., K. Jasniewicz, B. Meczekalski, et al. Polymorphic variants of genes encoding MTHFR, MTR, and MTHFD1 and the risk of depression in postmenopausal women in Poland. *Maturitas.* (2008) 61(3): 252-55.

4. Lewandowska, J., A. Bartoszek. DNA methylation in cancer development, diagnosis and therapy—multiple opportunities for genotoxic agents to act as methylome disruptors or remediators. *Mutagenesis.* (2011) 26(4): 475-87.

5. Douaud, G., H. Refsum, C.A. de Jager, et al. Preventing Alzheimer's disease-related gray matter atrophy by B-vitamin treatment. *Proceedings of the National Academy of Sciences* (2013) 110(23): 9523-28.

6. Werner, P., A. Di Rocco, A. Prikhojan, et al. COMT-dependent protection of dopaminergic neurons by methionine, dimethionine and S-adenosylmethionine (SAM) against L-dopa toxicity in vitro. *Brain research* (2001) 893(1): 278-81.

7. Zoccolella, S., S. V. Lamberti, G. Iliceto, et al. Hyperhomocysteinemia in l-dopa treated patients with Parkinson's disease: potential implications in cognitive dysfunction and dementia? *Current medicinal chemistry* (2010) 17(28): 3253-61.

8. Lipton, B. *The Biology of Belief: Unleashing the Power of Consciousness, Matter & Miracles.* Santa Rosa, CA: Elite Books (2005).

9. NIH National Human Genome Research Institute. A Brief History of the Human Genome Project. www.genome.gov/12011239/a-brief-history-of-the-human-genome-project/ Accessed January 2, 2017.

10. Spencer, M.D., T.J. Hamp, R.W. Reid, et al. Association between composition of the human gastrointestinal microbiome and development of fatty liver with choline deficiency. *Gastroenterology.* (2011) 140(3): 976-86.

11. Pacana, T., S. Cazanave, A. Verdianelli, et al. Dysregulated hepatic methionine metabolism drives homocysteine elevation in diet-induced nonalcoholic fatty liver disease. *PloS one.* (2015) 10(8): e0136822.

12. Kwon, D.Y., Y.S. Jung, S.J. Kim, et al. Impaired sulfur-amino acid metabolism and oxidative stress in nonalcoholic fatty liver are alleviated by betaine supplementation in rats. *The Journal of Nutrition.* (2009) 139(1): 63-68.

13. Pooya, S., S. Blaise, M.M. Garcia, et al. Methyl donor deficiency impairs fatty acid oxidation through PGC-1α hypomethylation and decreased ER-α, ERR-α, and HNF-4α in the rat liver. *Journal*

of Hepatology. (2012) 57(2): 344–51.

14. Dahlhoff, C., S. Worsch, M. Sailer, et al. Methyl-donor supplementation in obese mice prevents the progression of NAFLD, activates AMPK and decreases acyl-carnitine levels. *Molecular metabolism.* (2014) 3(5): 565–80.

15. Definition of haplotype/haplotypes. Scitable web page. www.nature.com/scitable/definition/haplotype-haplotypes-142. Accessed January 2, 2017.

4.

_____

HEALTH BEGINS IN THE STOMACH

Science never solves a problem without creating 10 more.

—George Bernard Shaw

Have you ever heard that we eat first with our eyes? It's true! The sight of food activates a series of neurological reflexes and pathways that primes our system for digestion. Unfortunately, just looking at food is not enough to digest it; we actually need to get all those nutrients inside our body. Most people assume that if they chew food and swallow it, they will absorb it, but this is not always the case. To experience abundant, lasting, radiant health, we have to make sure our gut is healthy. And in today's hectic, stressed-out world, most people are lacking in the digestion department.

What we digest, rather than what we put into our mouths, has everything to do with what we absorb. Eating your veggies is a good thing, but making sure they are fully absorbed is something different entirely. These nuances of digestion will become clear when we look at how the stomach actually functions in day-to-day life.

The process of digestion is very complex and requires a lot of energy—more than almost any other function of our body. With the body requiring high energy every day, its digestive system becomes an easy target when we start dealing with long-term health issues. The reason we suffer from poor digestion is because stress, toxins, malnutrition, and lack of bowel movement conspire to interfere with this most important process. And genetic imbalances certainly don't help.

Methylation problems make digestion more difficult for multiple reasons. When genetic pathways that produce energy, DNA, RNA, and antioxidants aren't working well, our stomach becomes one of the first organs that shuts down. Why would the body waste energy on producing acids and enzymes to digest food if it doesn't have enough energy for detoxification, cell repair, and immune defense?

The body is perfect at prioritizing; it will shut down stomach acid production to save that energy for something it knows is more life-critical at that moment, such as fueling the heart and brain. But that isn't health—that's just surviving. And we are interested in thriving!

THE ACID REFLUX PARADOX

Compared to an organ like the brain, the stomach is very simple, but the stomach's simple design doesn't protect it from dysfunction. Stomach problems are among the most common complaints in American society. It is estimated that up to 80 million Americans suffer from gastroesophageal reflux disease (GERD).[1] And sales of the acid-blocking proton-pump inhibitor Nexium (aka the purple pill) are in excess of $6 billion per year, making it the second highest selling drug in America.[2] If 25 percent of the population suffers from acid reflux, and acid-blocker manufacturers are selling billions of dollars of product each year, it's obvious that people are dealing with a lot of stomach problems! Of course, it doesn't have to be that way. The tools provided in this book can help make huge improvements in your digestion without resorting to dangerous drugs or treatments. You will find solutions throughout the protocol sections in this

SNPs of Concern

ACE/AGT/ADD1: These genes cause an increase in the angiotensin hormone. This hormone is released when we go into "fight-or-flight" stress. It causes blood vessels to constrict, raising blood pressure. This is why people are prescribed ACE-inhibitor medications to try and block this hormone. The ACE/AGT/ADD1 genes cause the blood vessels in the gut to constrict, lowering blood flow and oxygen to the tissues. This leads to less stomach acid being produced and increases the risk of ulcers and gastritis as well.

COMT/MAO: These genes increase effects of stress and adrenaline, which also reduce blood flow to the gut similar to angiotensin.

book; for now, though, let's keep learning about how your body's genius digestive system works, starting with the stomach.

The stomach's main job is to produce an acidic digestive juice, hydrochloric acid (HCl). When the stomach is working normally, this stomach acid should reach a pH of around 3.0. To make the acid that the stomach depends on for proper digestion, an enormous amount of energy is required—in fact, it takes about 1500 calories per day to produce sufficient stomach acid.[3] And these calories have to come from the mitochondria located in the stomach. When we are tired, toxic, sleep-deprived, or suffering from any number of chronic conditions, the body will struggle to produce enough cellular energy, and the stomach acid levels will decline. People suffering from untreated methylation issues are clearly at risk for low stomach acid, because methylation issues significantly impact the function of mitochondria.

Low stomach acid leads to other issues: it is a risk for bacterial overgrowth, and without sufficient acid in the stomach, the environment in the small intestine changes and the pancreas and the gallbladder are unable to release their digestive juices. Normally, the pancreas releases enzymes and bicarbonates that help digest food and raise the pH of the small intestine. When the stomach acid is absent, the pancreatic juices are absent. This is why laboratory testing of patients with irritable bowel syndrome (IBS) and other gut problems routinely show low elastase (an enzyme that breaks down proteins) and an acidic pH; these are two consequences of the pancreas and gallbladder not releasing digestive juices and one of many examples of how shutting off stomach acid by taking acid-blocking drugs greatly disrupts the digestive process.

Without the energy necessary to create sufficient quantities of stomach acid, our digestion slows down and we will likely suffer from leaky gut and poor digestion. In addition, deficiencies in folate, B12, choline, TMG, and betaine (each an important methyl donor) will lower the enzyme speed of our methyl cycle, which is like trying to run errands all over town in a car stuck in second gear. Low stomach acid is a big reason why people with methylation problems are riddled with digestive issues!

The critical point here is that stomach problems, especially problems with heartburn and acid reflux, have more to do with too little acid rather than too much. The vast majority of stomach problems result from too little acid in the stomach! This might seem counterintuitive, and it's a point that has caused a great deal of confusion, even among doctors. It is quite the paradox that low stomach acid can be responsible for acid reflux and GERD and doesn't make sense—until you understand how acid helps the stomach work effectively.

YOUR STOMACH: THE MUSCULAR OVEN

Think of the stomach as a muscular bag that acts like an oven, helping us cook our food by creating an acidic environment that breaks down our meals and releases nutrients. Like all ovens, the stomach must reach a certain temperature—or in this case, a certain acidity—in order to cook the food properly. If the door to the oven cannot close all the way, or if the oven cannot reach a high enough temperature, the food will be ruined and will not get cooked.

If the lower and upper sphincters in the stomach do not work correctly, the acid in the stomach will not stay where it should. And if the stomach is unable to make enough stomach acid, the stomach pH rises, it becomes too alkaline, and digestion decreases. Healthy digestion, as you shall see, is really all about making enough acid.

The hydrochloric acid in the stomach starts the process of breaking down the food we consume. A large amount of stomach acid creates an environment with a low pH, which turns on enzymes called proteases that break up protein bonds necessary for digestion. The digestive process continues from the stomach down through the small and large intestines, where nutrition that sustains our body is absorbed.

Although most people's stomachs don't make enough acid, some uncommon situations cause the body to make too much. For example, a rare tumor can grow in the small intestine near the stomach and cause copious amounts of stomach acid to be produced. This can lead to ulcers and internal bleeding. This cancer and a few other uncommon issues are the only health conditions that exist that cause too much acid. Just about everything else, including methylation imbalances, fatigue, poor sleep, over-consumption of processed food, mold and toxin exposure, and autoimmune conditions, make it harder for the body to make enough stomach acid. And this is by far our biggest threat to our digestive health.

Let's assume for the moment that you are experiencing heartburn. You feel a burning sensation in your upper chest, and the back of your throat feels itchy, tingles, and tastes acidic. You might even taste your meal hours after you finished eating it—yuck! And if you are to believe what you see on television and in magazine ads, your next step should be to go grab a TUMS, Zantac, or Nexium to make your acid reflux go away.

If those over-the-counter meds don't stop the pain, you may even visit your doctor for a prescription proton-pump inhibitor. And if you did take any of these med-

Conditions Associated with Stomach Acid Production

Insufficient stomach acid causes a large number of problems and diseases that affect our bones, brains, and immune systems:

- *burping*
- *hiccups*
- *acid reflux*
- *foul breath*
- *GERD*
- *foul smelling stools*
- *low B_{12}/B_9*
- *anemia*
- *osteoporosis*
- *leaky gut syndrome*
- *gallbladder disease*
- *adrenal fatigue*
- *methylation imbalances*
- *gut infections*
- *chronic fatigue*
- *fibromyalgia*
- *multiple chemical sensitivity disorder*

  Excess stomach acid can cause the following, less common conditions:
- *ulcers*
- *gastritis*
- *cancer, such as Zollinger-Ellison syndrome*

ications, your acid reflux would go away. However, your symptoms would disappear not because you fixed the problem, but because the drugs covered it up. These symptoms are necessary, however; they tell you what is wrong and offer direction as to how to fix the problem. And shouldn't that be the focus of your efforts to get healthy?

The main source of pain from acid reflux and heartburn is a sensation from the lining of the esophagus. This lining isn't as robust and thick as the stomach lining, and when acidic contents leave the stomach and "spill" up into the esophagus, it can irritate and damage this lining. If this happens once in a while, the body can easily recover. However, if heartburn and re-flux become chronic problems, damage to the esophagus can become so extreme that cancer may result.[4] This esophageal cancer, called Barrett's esophagus, is a direct result of the chronic inflammation caused by stom-ach acid irritating the esophagus. But fear not, because Barrett's esopha-gus is entirely preventable by implementing the genius body strategies discussed here for healthy stomach function. Even if someone already has esophageal damage, fixing the issues in the stomach will enable the esophagus to heal.

At this juncture, let's consider a question: If food is supposed to go from the esophagus into the stomach, what causes it to go back from the stom-ach into the esophagus? The answer has to do with the function of the sphincter, or "oven door," that controls food entering the stomach from the esophagus. As you can see in Figure 4.1, the stomach is designed with two doors, or sphincters: the lower esophageal sphincter (LES) between the esophagus and the stomach and the pyloric sphincter (PS) between the stomach and the intestines.

The LES has to relax to allow food coming from the mouth to enter the stomach. Once food enters the stomach, the LES contracts and closes to keep the food inside for proper digestion to occur. If this sphincter doesn't close all the way, some of the food and gastric juices will flow up into the esophagus. This causes pain and is the root cause of all heartburn. Lucky for us, the body has a genius method for preventing food from leaving the stomach upward instead of moving downward like it should.

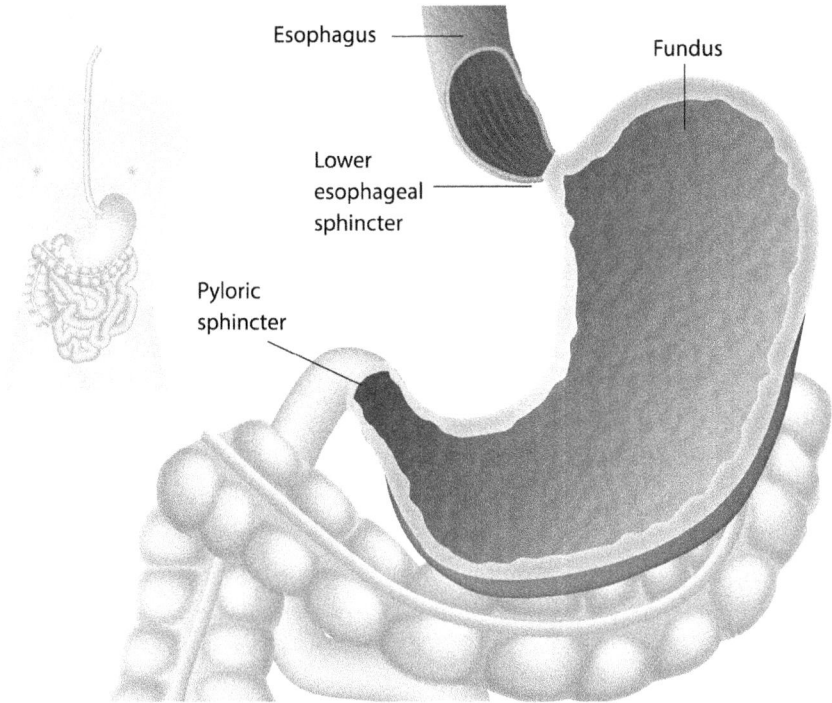

Figure 4.1 - *Anatomy of the stomach showing the lower esophageal sphincter and pyloric sphincter*

Here's the body's genius trick for preventing heartburn: When the acidic gastric juice produced in the stomach splashes onto the LES, it causes the sphincter to contract and close tight. Research has shown that when the stomach contents reach a pH of 3.0 (very acidic), the LES is fully closed.[5] The large amount of hydrochloric acid in the stomach, which is a normal and healthy part of digestion, actually prevents GERD (heartburn or reflux) by tightening the LES and preventing the acid from splashing into the esophagus.[6]

We experience heartburn when the LES doesn't function correctly and acid escapes from the stomach and splashes up into the esophagus. When this acidic, partially digested food exits the stomach, it inflames the lining of the throat and esophagus, and this is where the pain from GERD comes from. However, even though the undigested food leaving the stomach is acidic and hurts the esophagus, it is still not acidic enough in terms of a healthy stomach. Allow me to explain this further:

- Food enters the stomach and mixes with gastric juices (hydrochloric acid).

- The pH of this mixture should be around 3.0, which is perfect for the stomach to start breaking down proteins and other molecules. However, because of hectic modern lifestyles, poor sleep, toxins, food allergies, and poor eating habits, most people do not produce enough stomach acid, and their stomach pH is higher, or more alkaline, than it should be.

- With inadequate acidity in the stomach (a pH higher than 3.0), the lower esophageal sphincter will not close all the way and remains partially open. Remember that the LES closes when the pH reaches 3.0.

- As the muscles of the stomach swish food around during digestion, some acid from the stomach can splash up onto the esophagus, causing pain—OUCH!

When stomach acid creates a pH of 3.0, heartburn and reflux are prevented because the LES is tightly closed. A pH of 4 or 5 is still acidic in terms of the esophagus and will burn the lining of the esophagus and throat, but as far as the stomach is concerned, it is not acidic enough for optimal stomach and LES function. In a nutshell, when there's not enough acid to activate the LES, the sphincter stays open and acid splashes up and burns your throat.

The sad part is that although we've known about this phenomenon for the last 45 years, the scientific proof doesn't seem to be persuasive enough to change the way many doctors treat patients who suffer with GERD.

HIATAL HERNIAS AND ACID REFLUX

Another important part of the heartburn issue is the hiatal hernia. A hiatal hernia is a problem that occurs when the upper part of the stomach slides up into the diaphragm, distorting the shape of the stomach and esophagus (Figure 4.2). These stomach hernias slow down peristalsis–the rhythmic contraction of muscle that helps move food from our mouth to our stomach–and make it more difficult for the LES of the stomach to close properly.[7, 8] Hiatal hernias make it more difficult for food to reach the stomach and stay there once it arrives. And it makes it difficult to swallow food and predisposes us to heartburn, GERD, and even heart arrhythmia.

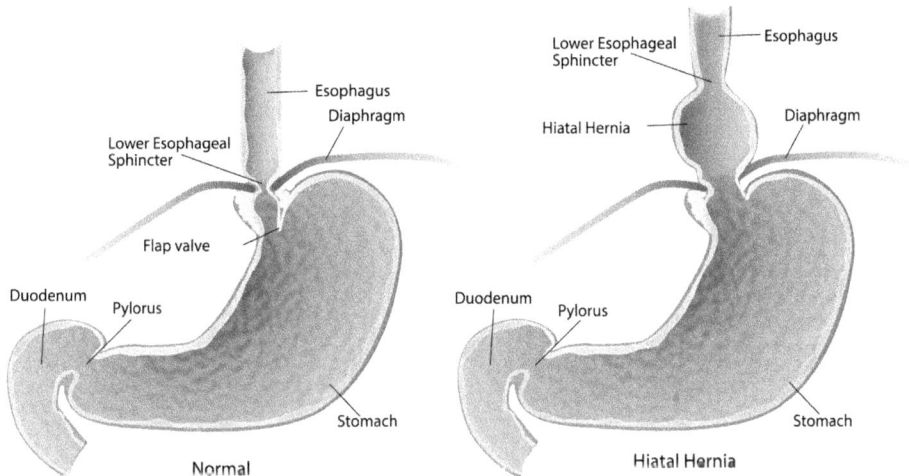

Figure 4.2 - *Stomach anatomy and hiatal hernia, showing stomach pushed up into the diaphragm on the image at right*

You don't need expensive, invasive, and possibly dangerous endoscopy studies to determine whether you have a hiatal hernia. Although those specialized medical procedures are capable of diagnosing this condition, there is a better way: Look at the heart instead of the stomach. Because of the anatomical position of the stomach when it slides up into the diaphragm, it can rub against and squeeze the heart. When this happens, patients often experience arrhythmia or palpitations after eating, and especially when they lie down or try to sleep. Studies show that those who have a hiatal hernia are 21 times (2100 percent) more likely to have arrhythmia or heart palpitations, due largely to mechanical pressure of the stomach against the heart.[9, 10] This knowledge has served me well, and I now assume everyone with arrhythmia has a hiatal hernia until proven otherwise. I am not a betting man, but 21:1 are pretty good odds that folks suffering with arrhythmia have undiagnosed and untreated hiatal hernias!

Occasionally, a hiatal hernia can be a serious medical problem that requires surgery. However, most hiatal hernias are not quite bad enough for surgery but are not quite working optimally either. Regardless, a hiatal hernia interferes with the function of the stomach, making it harder for food to get into the stomach and harder to keep it there once it arrives. This is why a hiatal hernia can be a big player in causing heartburn.

When we suffer from poor stomach function or a hiatal hernia, we need to look at all the factors involved, and without a doubt, the health of the diaphragm is at the top of that list. Many people with a hiatal hernia, and GERD or reflux in general, also have a weak diaphragm. Like any muscle in the body, the diaphragm can become weak over time, especially for those who have poor posture, who lack exercise, or who have joint problems in the neck or back. Like many problems in the body, a weak diaphragm can go unnoticed for weeks, months, or years—the only symptom being chronic acid reflux.

Because the diaphragm and the stomach sit together anatomically, they are linked together in their structure and function. The shape of the diaphragm helps prevent the stomach from sliding up and creating a hiatal hernia. And when the diaphragm is strong and functioning correctly, the tension in the diaphragm muscle helps to keep the LES working optimally.

To determine whether acid reflux is caused by a weak diaphragm, you need to test diaphragm function accurately. The best tools for this include a peak flow meter, an oxygen saturation device, and manual muscle testing through the use of applied kinesiology—all things I use regularly to help my patients. (I would encourage anyone dealing with acid reflux to seek out a chiropractor in their area who is trained in applied kinesiology. For more information on applied kinesiology and finding a doctor in your area who is certified in this specialty, see the appendix.)

CHRONIC PROBLEMS CAUSED BY INSUFFICIENT STOMACH ACID AND PPIS

At this point, you realize that heartburn is caused by too little acid in the stomach and an upper stomach sphincter that cannot close properly. But what happens to the body when the stomach cannot produce enough acid? Insufficient stomach acid can create some serious, potentially life-threatening problems down the road. Sounds extreme, but keep reading and you'll see why.

To treat stomach complaints, the American healthcare system relies heavily on expensive drugs and over-the-counter (OTC) acid-blockers that make the symptoms go away. This type of approach has generated a lot of research that helps us understand what happens when the stomach stops producing hydrochloric acid for digestion. Because tens of millions of Americans are taking some kind of acid-blocking medication, we are beginning to see the long-term effects of these drugs. And, dear reader, it is not a pretty picture. Truth is, taking prescription and OTC acid-blockers long term greatly increases the risk for problems much bigger than either heartburn or indigestion.

The most powerful antacid drugs, proton-pump inhibitors (PPIs), shut down the ability of the acid-producing cells in the stomach to produce acid. They make heartburn go away, but they also stop the stomach from digesting food. We now know that giving PPI drugs to people without heartburn will actually cause them to have heartburn when they stop taking the drug! In a 2009 study, PPI drugs were taken by healthy individuals who did not suffer from reflux. After eight weeks, they stopped taking the drugs, and about half the participants developed acid reflux symptoms.[11] When we create drugs to stop normal, physiological processes inside the body, the body often produces a counter-reaction. What we call "side effects" are often just attempts by the body to overcome the toxic effects of the medication.

When medical researchers compared the stomachs of those suffering from peptic ulcers and reflux against those who had no stomach problems, they found something interesting: Patients who had ulcer and reflux problems also had lower stomach acid on average (meaning a higher, or more alkaline, stomach pH) and more bile fluid inside the stomach.[12] This contradicts the idea that ulcers and other stomach conditions are caused by too much acid. In reality, the majority of these stomach conditions are associated with too little stomach acid, not too much. Only in rare cases are ulcers caused by the production of too much acid. One such rare situation is Zollinger-Ellison syndrome, caused by a gastrin-secreting tumor that produces excessive acid, leading to ulcer formation.[13]

For the vast majority of people who suffer from ulcers, the mucosal defenses of the stomach are shut down, so that whatever acid is present can easily burn and injure the stomach lining. It is important to point out that NSAID drugs such as ibuprofen and naproxen actually set the stage for ulcers to form in the first place. These commonly used, "harmless" drugs cause holes to develop in the protective mucous layer of the stomach, leading to gastritis and life-threatening bleeding ulcers.[14] And how many people take these medications every day? Millions upon millions! Even aspirin, that seemingly harmless medication widely used to treat heart disease, can cause serious bleeding problems in the upper GI tract. In fact, even a low dose of just 10 mg per day of aspirin causes significant injury to the stomach lining.[15] Unfortunately, many people take low doses of aspirin for years on end, likely oblivious to the ongoing damage it causes in their stomach and intestines.

You can see just how important stomach acid really is by looking at what happens when there isn't enough of it. In other words, when you don't make enough stomach acid, major problems will arise in other parts of your body. As the research illustrates, the longer we live with low stomach acid, the bigger the problems we face.

An important study published in the *Journal of the American Medical Association* in 2006 shed light on this issue by concluding that long-term PPI usage actually increased the risk of hip fracture.[16] Without sufficient stomach acid, the body has a more difficult time absorbing calcium and other minerals that strengthen bones, because these molecules require an acidic environment to be fully digested. People who take acid-blockers short- or long-term are jeopardizing their bone health. This fact was confirmed in a later study published in 2009, which showed that low stomach acid, aka hypochlorhydria, is a risk factor for osteoporosis.[17] These studies provide convincing evidence that proper stomach function is a prerequisite for bone health as we age.

It is clear by now that low stomach acid reduces calcium absorption, and low calcium absorption leads to bone loss over time. Unfortunately, the problems caused by acid-blocking drugs and hypochlorhydria (a deficiency of stomach acids) don't stop with weakening our bones. The truth is, issues caused by low stomach function will affect many other bodily tissues. A recent study published in the *American Journal of Gastroenterology* points out that in addition to hip fracture (osteoporosis), long-term PPI use can cause *Clostridium difficile*, a serious gut bug that is associated with diarrhea, pneumonia, vitamin B12 deficiency, and even death in severe cases.[18] And brand new studies now prove that PPI drugs cause damage to the kidneys and the brain, two of our most sensitive organs.

A groundbreaking study released early in 2016 in the prestigious journal *JAMA Neurology* connects the dots between PPI use and Alzheimer's disease. The researchers looked at more than 73,000 patients and discovered that PPI use after age 75 increased the risk of Alzheimer's by 50 percent.[19] Another study released early in 2016 in the journal *JAMA Internal Medicine* warns that PPI use also increases the risk of chronic kidney disease by 50 percent.[20] So use of PPIs might make your heartburn go away, but you could suffer serious chronic disease down the road as a result. You will likely not feel that pain in your esophagus, but you will be at an increased risk for pneumonia, gut infections, dementia, and other widespread biochemical issues stemming from a lack of vitamin B12. That, my friend, is a very poor tradeoff.

Although these powerful drugs are routinely given to children and infants, the most sensitive population taking these drugs is the elderly. Since stomach function declines with age, giving an elderly person an acid-blocking drug will dramatically reduce his or her ability to get nutrition from food. And although children and infants who are given these drugs may use them for a short period, seniors and adults who are prescribed these toxic meds often take them for years, even decades.

How can acid-blocking drugs cause symptoms as varied as diarrhea, pneumonia, osteoporosis, and neurological decline from low B12 levels? The answer lies in realizing that low stomach acid allows bad bacteria from the gut to crawl up into the small intestine and pass through the stomach. When we are sleeping, we can inhale this gut-derived bacteria as it crawls headward, leading to lung infections and pneumonia. When we are healthy, our stomach acid acts like an acid-bath that prevents bugs in our gut from crawling uphill and prevents bugs in the food we eat from making us ill. I'll bet you never thought about that when you last reached for a bottle of acid-blocking pills.

It is well known that shutting down stomach function makes it difficult for the body to absorb vitamins, especially critical ones like B12 and vitamin D. We can see how the elderly are vulnerable by looking again at recent research on B12 deficiency. A study published in 2008 illustrates how long-term PPI therapy causes B12 deficiency in older adults, even if they are taking the RDA recommended amount of B12 in their diet.[21] The aging body already has a hard time absorbing vitamins, so anything that gets in the way of stomach acid production will worsen the low-absorption problem. These acid-blocking drugs shut down parietal cells that make both stomach acid and intrinsic factor, a protein that is absolutely required for our bodies to absorb B12 from our diet. When we take a drug that interferes with intrinsic factor production, it stops us from being able to absorb the incredibly powerful B12 vitamin. That leads over time to a decrease in vitamin B12 levels, resulting in neurological degeneration, anemia, and even death. [22]

Finally, current research also confirms that lack of stomach acid from PPI drug use can cause dangerously low levels of critical minerals such as magnesium, calcium, potassium, and sodium.[23, 24] And all this from a medication widely considered to be safe and well-tolerated.

The bottom line with acid-blocking drugs is that they are a recipe for health problems ranging from malnutrition, to osteoporosis, to chronic gut infections. Without sufficient production of stomach acid, the pancreas and gallbladder will not release digestive juices, and this makes it very difficult for the body to absorb vitamins. Stomach acid is so critical for the process of absorption that shutting it down will make it nearly impossible to get all the nutrients we need from our diet.

CONCLUSION

If there is a single root cause of chronic illness, it has to be poor digestion. Living with poor stomach function means living in a state of less optimum health. And because stomach function is the keystone to health, interfering with stomach acid production is a dangerous game that leads to numerous chronic health problems. This chapter exposed the causes of heartburn and reflux, along with the dark side of acid-blocking drugs. Knowing this information gives you a better understanding about why we experience heartburn, and knowledge leads to power and good health. And shouldn't that be what doctors teach their patients? Given all the problems with these medications, it is no wonder that people who take these drugs regularly struggle to get healthy—for without a healthy gut, it is impossible to have a healthy body. How can the body heal if the medications we take stop our digestive process from working?

My patients often hear me say that the body never makes mistakes—the body is a genius. We may think that our body isn't working when we experience heartburn (or any health problem, for that matter), when in fact the body is always acting correctly given the circumstances. We can take supplements to support and heal the stomach, change our eating habits, better manage our stress, and work with a chiropractor or natural medicine doctor with the skills to treat GERD or a hiatal hernia and strengthen the diaphragm. This approach takes more work and time than popping a pill, but it also rewards you with positive life-enhancing side effects instead of toxic, health-destroying ones. To me, this is a no-brainer!

Now that you understand the issues that occur with poor stomach function, let's take a step farther into the body and learn about another potential pitfall. In the next chapter, we'll uncover the story of oxalates, a gut-based toxin that can have major impacts on our kidneys, liver, brain, and methylation cycle in general.

STOMACH PROTOCOL

The best way to support proper stomach function is to make sure there is enough acid in the stomach. Since everyone is different, there is no single dose that is best for all patients. To determine how much betaine hydrochloride is required for an individual, a dosing experiment called the HCl Challenge is used. You can find more about the HCl Challenge in appendix D. For those individuals with an inflamed stomach lining who cannot tolerate stomach acid supplements, I have shared a gastritis repair protocol that can greatly reduce the pain and burning in the stomach and esophagus.

RECOMMENDED LAB TESTING:

I recommend the Routine Blood Tests and the Organic Acid Test in appendix B for assessing the gut, brain, mitochondria, and other factors. To make full use of the information in this book I recommend following the instructions in appendix A to get your own detailed genetic report.

LOW STOMACH ACID PROTOCOL:

HCl Support – HCl stomach acid that will support the digestion and break down of your food. Take this product right at the end of the meal. To find out what dose is best for you, see the HCl stomach acid instructions page.† (Nutridyn)

Pan 5X – Pancreatic enzymes that will help you break down your food. Take 1 or 2 tablets five minutes before meals/shakes/snacks. Will improve digestion and absorption of nutrients.† (Nutridyn)

NOTE: If pain or discomfort occurs when taking HCl Support, it indicates inflammation of the lining of the stomach and esophagus. To heal the stomach and esophagus, use the Gastritis Repair Protocol that follows for at least 4 weeks before trying to reintroduce the HCl Support.

GASTRITIS AND ULCER REPAIR PROTOCOL:

This protocol is for those individuals who have active gastritis, who cannot tolerate stomach acid supplements at any dose, or who are healing from an *H. pylori* infection. The following protocol should be taken for at least 4 weeks. After one month, the dosages may be reduced and the supplements can be taken long term for ongoing support as needed.

Dynamic GI Integrity – Mix 1/2 scoop into water 6 times per day. Take it immediately after each meal, making sure to take at least one serving every 2-3 hours. Powerful support that will help reduce inflammation of the upper GI tract. Acts as a calming salve to relieve burning pain associated with gastritis and inflammation of the mucosa.†* (Nutridyn)

Zinc-Carnosine – 1 capsuless 2 times per day away from food. Zinc-carnosine will enhance the repair of the stomach lining; used in Japan for decades to repair gastric mucosa after antibiotic therapy.† (Nutridyn)

†This statement has not been evaluated by the FDA. This product is not intended to diagnose, treat, cure, or prevent any disease. The information provided in this book is intended for your general knowledge only and is not a substitute for professional medical advice or treatment for specific medical conditions. You should not use this information to diagnose or treat a health problem or disease without consulting with a qualified healthcare provider. Please consult your healthcare provider with any questions or concerns you may have regarding your condition. Never disregard professional medical advice or delay in seeking it because of something you have read in this book.

REFERENCES

1. El-Serag, H.B., S. Sweet, C.C. Winchester, et al. Update on the epidemiology of gastroesophageal reflux disease: a systematic review. *Gut.* (2013). [Epub ahead of print]

2. DeNoon, D.J. "The 10 Most Prescribed Drugs." WebMD Health News. www.webmd. com/news/20110420/the-10-most-prescribed-drugs. Published April 20, 2011. Accessed January 7, 2016.

3. Guyton, A.C., J.E. Hall. *Textbook of Medical Physiology*, 11th ed. Philadelphia, PA: Elsevier (2006) p. 796.

4. Taylor, J.B., J.H. Rubenstein. Meta-analyses of the effect of symptoms of gastroesophageal reflux on the risk of Barrett's esophagus. *Am J Gastroenterol.* (2010) 105(8): 1729, 1730-37; quiz 1738.

5. Giles, G.R., C. Humphries, M.C. Mason, et al. Effect of pH changes on the cardiac sphincter. *Gut.* (1969) 10(10): 852-56.

6. Sandler, A.D., J.F. Schlegel, J.W. Maher, et al. The mechanism of acid-induced increases in canine lower esophageal sphincter pressure. *Surgery.* (1989) 105(4): 529-34.

7. Roman, S., P.J. Kahrilas, L. Kia, et al. Effects of large hiatal hernias on esophageal peristalsis. *Arch Surg.* (2012) 147(4): 352-57.

8. Hirsch, D.P., G.N. Tytgat, G.E. Boeckxstaens. Transient lower esophageal sphincter relaxations—a pharmacological target for gastroesophageal reflux disease? *Aliment Pharmacol Ther.* (2002) 16(1): 17-26.

9. Roman, C., S. Bruley des Varannes, L. Muresan, et al. Atrial fibrillation in patients with gastroesophageal reflux disease: a comprehensive review. *World J Gastroenterol.* (2014) 20(28): 9592-99.

10. Roy, R.R., S. Sagar, T.J. Bunch, et al. Hiatal Hernia is associated with an increased prevalence of atrial fibrillation in young patients. *Hypertension.* (2013) 49: 40.

11. Reimer, C., B. Søndergaard, L. Hilsted, et al. Proton-pump inhibitor therapy induces acid-related symptoms in healthy volunteers after withdrawal of therapy. *Gastroenterology.* (2009) 137(1): 80-87.

12. Dixon, M.F., H.J. O'Connor, A.T. Axon, et al. Reflux gastritis: distinct histopathological entity? *J Clin Pathol.* (1986) 39(5): 524-30.

13. Riff, B.P., D.A. Leiman, B. Bennett, et al. Weight Gain in Zollinger-Ellison Syndrome After Acid Suppression. *Pancreas.* (2015). [Epub ahead of print]. Accessed January 7, 2016.

14. Castellsague, J., N. Riera-Guardia, B. Calingaert, et al. Individual NSAIDs and upper gastrointestinal complications: a systematic review and meta-analysis of observational studies (the SOS project). *Drug Saf.* (2012) 35(12): 1127-46.

15. Iwamoto, J., Y. Saito, A. Honda, et al. Clinical features of gastroduodenal injury associated with long-term low-dose aspirin therapy. *World J Gastroenterol*. (2013) 19(11): 1673-82.

16. Yang, Y.X., J.D. Lewis, S. Epstein, et al. Long-term proton pump inhibitor therapy and risk of hip fracture. *JAMA*. (2006) 296(24): 2947-53.

17. Schinke, T., A.F. Schilling, A. Baranowsky, et al. Impaired gastric acidification negatively affects calcium homeostasis and bone mass. *Nat Med*. (2009) 15(6): 674-81.

18. Heidelbaugh, J.J., K.L. Goldberg, J.M. Inadomi. Overutilization of proton pump inhibitors: a review of cost-effectiveness and risk [corrected]. *Am J Gastroenterol*. (2009) 104 Suppl 2: S27-32.

19. Gomm, W., K. von Holt, F. Thomé, et al. Association of Proton Pump Inhibitors with Risk of Dementia: A Pharmacoepidemiological Claims Data Analysis. *JAMA Neurol*. (2016) **73(4): 410-16.**

20. Lazarus, B., Y. Chen, F.P. Wilson, et al. Proton Pump Inhibitor Use and the Risk of Chronic Kidney Disease. *JAMA Intern Med*. (2016) 176(2): 238-46.

21. O Dharmarajan, T.S., M.R. Kanagala, P. Murakonda, et al. Do acid-lowering agents affect vitamin B12 status in older adults? *J Am Med Dir Assoc*. (2008) 9(3): 162-67.

22. Festen, H.P. Intrinsic factor secretion and cobalamin absorption. Physiology and pathophysiology in the gastrointestinal tract. *Scand J Gastroenterol Suppl*. (1991) 188: 1-7.

23. Gouraud, A., V. Vochelle, J. Descotes, et al. Proton pump inhibitor-induced neutropenia: possible cross-reactivity between omeprazole and pantoprazole. *Clin Drug Investig*. (2010) 30(8): 559-63.

24. Shabajee, N., E.J. Lamb, I. Sturgess, et al. Omeprazole and refractory hypomagnesaemia. *BMJ*. (2008) 337(7662): 173-75.

5.

THE OXALATE PROBLEM
YOU'VE NEVER HEARD OF

*The mind, once stretched by a new idea, never returns
to its original dimensions.*

—Ralph Waldo Emerson

No discussion of gut health and methylation would be complete without considering the problem of oxalates. Plants create oxalate crystals inside their cells as a self-defense mechanism to make themselves unpalatable to insect pests and grazing animals. Oxalates are like the thorns on a rose bush, except in this case, the thorns are hidden *on the inside* of the plant.

Foods that contain oxalates are some of the most common and healthiest foods we can eat: meat, coffee, chocolate, nuts and seeds, and many varieties of fruits and vegetables.[1,2] When we eat nutritious kale salads or drink spinach smoothies, we are getting the nutrients and antioxidants in those plants, but we are also getting the oxalates.

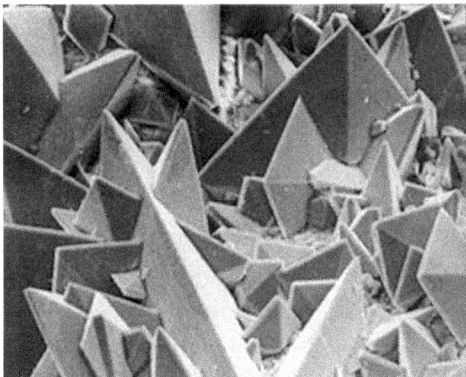

Figure 5.1 - Oxalates form microscopic crystals that resemble shards of glass. It isn't hard to imagine how these crystals can harm insects or cause pain inside our own tissues.

You may think that eating spinach, kale, and chard smoothies every day would do no harm! But what you might not realize is that by juicing every day, you may be overdosing on oxalates. It's not that these foods are bad for us, but as with many things in life, moderation is the key. Our body has the ability to manage mild levels of oxalates, but if oxalate levels build up too high, we are certain to suffer the consequences in our health and our genetic pathways.

The main reason oxalates become a problem is that they leak into the body through a dysfunctional gut and cause a wide range of health issues. Once inside, the oxalates tend to over-accumulate in our tissues and put strain on our kidneys. Most people first learn about oxalates after they suffer kidney stones—and an over-accumulation of oxalates causes about three-quarters of all such stones. Additionally, most of the research available comes from kidney doctors and nephrologists, which seems to suggest that the kidney is the only part of the body impacted by these plant toxins. Although kidney issues are the most well-known problems, oxalate issues can literally wreak havoc all over the body.

OXALATES AND LEAKY GUT

Although some rare genetic disorders cause a high amount of oxalates in the body, the vast majority of people with oxalate problems cannot blame it on their genes. In fact, most people develop oxalate problems because of poor digestion. And, without a doubt, a poorly functioning gallbladder is the number one reason for oxalate problems.

To illustrate the connection between gut dysfunction and oxalates, we can look at how oxalate levels rise in the body after bariatric surgery. Research has shown that individuals who compromise their upper GI tract with gastric bypass surgery develop hyperoxaluria—excess oxalates in the blood and urine.[3] The bariatric surgery-oxalate relationship is easy to understand. When we damage the stomach and gallbladder with an aggressive surgery, it begins to impair digestion, and as digestion becomes more dysfunctional, more oxalate problems develop. Simple as that.

As long as our digestion is working properly, producing stomach acid, and releasing enzymes and bile, the oxalates we consume in our food are not a problem. As long as our gallbladder is working well, we can eat food with oxalates and have no worries that we will develop an oxalate problem. The problem with oxalates arises because many of us don't have healthy gallbladder function.

Digestion should stimulate the release of bile from the gallbladder to digest fats in our diet and fend off the negative effects of oxalates. But many people suffer from terrible gallbladder function. Gallbladder surgery is still one of the most common surgeries in America, and oxalates build up and become a problem, especially for those with chronic gut or methylation issues.[4]

Bile acts like soap, chopping fat globules into tiny balls called micelles; this is necessary so that we can absorb all those healthy Omega 3 fats and fat-soluble vitamins such as A, D, E, and K. When the gallbladder is working properly, the fat in our diet is absorbed in the small intestine and the oxalates in our meal form a compound with calcium, calcium-oxalate, which we cannot absorb.[5] Bile helps us absorb the fats we need and pass the oxalates in our stool so they don't cause problems. Normally, our body will not absorb all calcium from food. As shown in Figure 5.2, the undigested calcium binds with the oxalates in the gut, which helps us to rid our body of this toxic molecule. However, this process slows down or ceases to occur when the gallbladder system begins to malfunction.

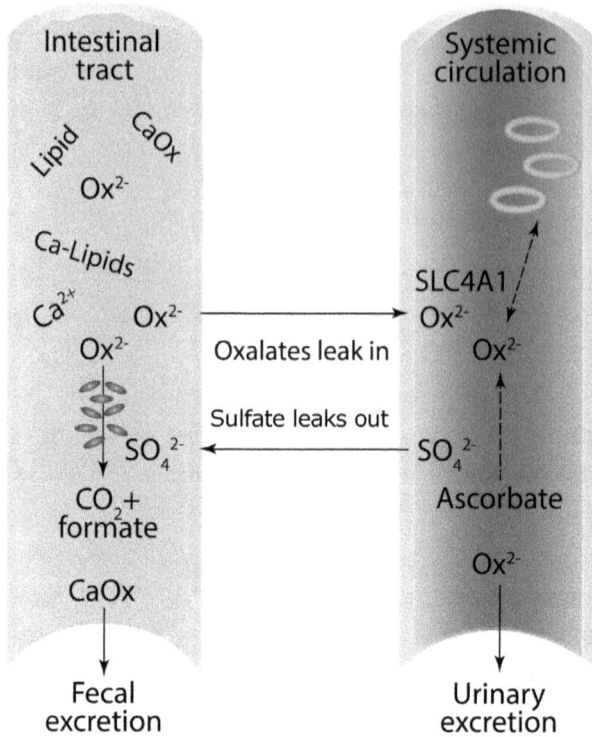

Figure 5.2 – *Oxalates are absorbed and produced inside the human body. Sulfate is lost into the intestines when oxalates leak in from our diet.*

When the gallbladder stops releasing bile, whether it is from stomach dysfunction, taurine deficiency, poor methylation, or some other health problem (such as having the gallbladder removed surgically), we absorb more oxalates. Without bile release, we cannot absorb fats. Since the fats are floating down the small intestine without being absorbed, they begin to bind with the calcium. When the fat isn't digested, the calcium attaches to the fats instead of the oxalates, which causes us to poop out all our healthy fats and calcium, leading to significant nutritional and health problems down the road, such as osteoporosis and inflammatory diseases. When we do not absorb fats properly, there is no calcium left to bind to the oxalates, and the body ends up absorbing high amounts of oxalates. And this causes problems in other parts of the body including the liver, kidneys, bladder, joints, muscles, and bones.

In a study released in 2015, researchers confirmed that not only do oxalates cause most kidney stones, but they also rob the body of calcium, leading to bone degeneration and osteoporosis.[6] When the gut cannot provide an adequate level of calcium for the rest of the body, the bones begin to deteriorate and release calcium into the bloodstream. If this happens for a long time, it results in hyperparathyroidism (which can lead to cancer and other serious health issues), bone loss, and osteoporosis. Too bad no one tells you that when you have your gallbladder removed!

CALCIUM AND KIDNEY PROBLEMS

The kidneys are especially sensitive to oxalates, which have a tendency to cause kidney stones. Not surprisingly, the latest research on kidney stones points clearly to problems in the gut as the root cause. Taking a closer look at the biochemical research, we can see clearly how oxalates, and by extension gut problems, are the most common causes of kidney stones.

Research published in the *New England Journal of Medicine* some 40 years ago shows the first indications that gut problems can cause oxalate issues in the kidneys. Researchers investigating ulcerative colitis patients found that after sections of the ileum (part of the small intestine) had been surgically removed, many individuals developed hyperoxaluria, an excessive urinary excretion of oxalate and a known risk factor for stone formation.[7] Later on, a study published in 2010 highlighted the fact that almost 75 percent of all kidney stones are in fact calcium-oxalate stones, further bolstering the connection between kidney damage and oxalate levels.[8] Both of these studies confirm that most people in the United States who have a kidney stone are actually suffering from an oxalate problem that starts in the gut!

You may have heard that excess calcium in the body can cause kidney stones. But we cannot blame calcium when the problem is caused by oxalates. As one of the most insoluble compounds in the body, oxalates hurt the kidneys and other tissues: if oxalate levels rise too high, they form crystals that are almost impossible for the body to dissolve.[9] These crystals can accumulate in the brain, lungs, blood vessels, joints, and bones, causing pain and dysfunction throughout the body.[10, 11, 12, 13] Oxalate crystals can be a hidden source of pain and dysfunction in dozens of chronic health problems ranging from autism, to fibromyalgia, to vulvodynia, interstitial cystitis, and more.

So if calcium-oxalate stones cause most kidney stones, should you avoid calcium in your diet? The answer is no! More calcium, not less, is needed in your diet if you want to prevent oxalate stones from forming. Although this sounds contradictory, the body has a genius reason for this. Research has proven that consuming more calcium will actually prevent calcium-oxalate stones by binding more of the oxalates in your gut.[14] Remember that oxalate kidney stones are really just a gut problem that shows up as a problem in the kidneys. In other words, when you fix the oxalate problem in the gut, you fix the oxalate problem in the kidneys.

To discourage oxalates from leaking into the gut, one of the best strategies is to take calcium-citrate before meals. This type of calcium does two things: First, it releases its calcium quickly into the gut, helping to bind up the extra oxalates floating around. Second, the citrate helps to prevent the calcium and the oxalate from binding inside the kidneys.[15, 16] That's a two-for-one that pays off! I routinely recommend this to my patients with excellent results. You'll find more specific information on how to heal oxalate problems with diet and supplements at the end of this chapter.

THE DOWNSIDE TO HIGH OXALATES: PROBLEMS WITH B6, SULFATE, GUT, AND METHYLATION

I wish I could stop here and say that I've covered all the damage that oxalates can do to the body, but that would fall short of capturing the full story. In addition to causing kidney stones and robbing us of calcium, healthy fats, and fat-soluble vitamins, oxalates also deplete the body's levels of sulfate and vitamin B6. These two nutrients are incredibly powerful and are absolutely necessary for our health and survival.

Remember that oxalates in mild amounts are not a problem; the body gets rid of oxalates by breaking them down in the liver and excreting them through the urine. As long as the body can safely detoxify oxalate molecules, they will not bother us. But one of the main reasons that oxalates are so toxic is that each oxalate molecule that gets into our body causes us to lose a molecule of sulfate.

Sulfate molecules are amazing; without this essential byproduct of our methylation cycle, we cannot survive. Sulfate helps us seal a leaky gut and strengthen the bones, ligaments, and tendons. It is required for phase II detoxification of all kinds of toxins, hormones, and heavy metals. In fact, sulfate is so important for our health that it is the fourth most common nutrient in the bloodstream![17]

Oxalates and sulfate use the same transporters to move through our bodies. On the surface of our gut, liver, and kidneys exists a cellular transporter called the Sat1 transport protein.[18] The job of this little cellular micro-machine is to exchange, or swap, one molecule of oxalate for one molecule of sulfate. It's like a revolving door that constantly pushes sulfate out in exchange for an oxalate molecule coming in. This Sat1 transporter works with a handful of other oxalate-sulfate exchangers to move sulfate into the gut or into the urine when our oxalate levels rise. You can see in Figure 5.3 a model of how this process works in our gut wall. The process in the kidneys is very similar.

SNPs of Concern

The genes most affected by oxalates will be the SULT and other Phase II-related pathways.

Phase II: A process where fat-soluble toxins are made water-soluble inside the liver and removed in the bile or urine.

SULT: The body's main Phase II detoxification enzyme, where a molecule of sulfur is glued to a toxin. Sulfur is sticky and oxalates cause sulfur deficiency, slowing down SULT. This forces the body to use other Phase II pathways, such as NAT, GSH, UGT, COMT, and MTHFR, which puts greater demand on these pathways, which are often genetically slowed down.

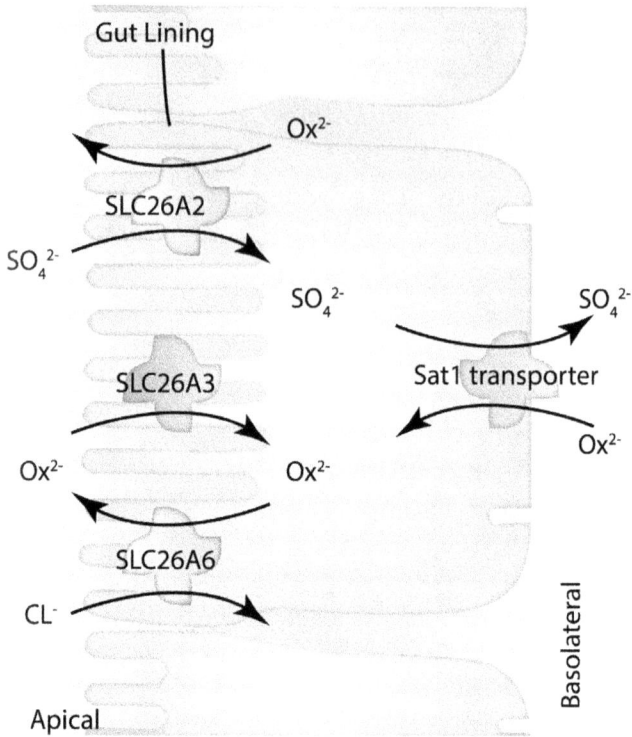

Figure 5.3 - *Sat1 and related transporters are found on cells lining the gut wall*

Imagine what happens when our gallbladder and digestion stop working well. A lot of oxalates from our diet make their way far down into the intestines to the colon. Here the oxalates are floating around and bumping into the gut wall. On the wall of our colon lives the Sat1 transporter, which grabs an oxalate molecule and drags it inside our body while simultaneously pumping out a sulfate molecule. Because we haven't digested our food well, we just lost a molecule we needed (sulfate) and gained one that causes problems (oxalate). If this happens once, it's no big deal; but you and I both know this would happen millions of times at the molecular level. I am confident the body has a genius reason for this—I just haven't figured this one out yet!

As our oxalate absorption increases, we begin to lose sulfate, and this carries serious consequences to our methylation cycle. The loss of sulfate into the gut and into the urine means the methylation cycle has to work harder to produce more sulfate, drawing down our nutrient savings account in an attempt to replace what is being lost. For our cells, this will cause more resources to be shifted toward detoxification and protection and fewer resources to be invested into growth and repair. Our cells will be stuck in fight or flight and won't be able to rest or digest very well—and neither will we.

Loss of sulfate can be challenging for the average person, and it can be an absolute disaster for someone with MTHFR, GST, GSS, GSR, SULT1A1, SULT2A1, and other polymorphisms. These individuals already have a slowed sulfate detoxification system, and any loss of sulfate can be devastating to their ability to build, repair, and detoxify. Individuals who have SULT SNPs are extra sensitive to low sulfate levels, because lack of sulfate exacerbates a slowed genetic pathway. Many people with SULT gene polymorphisms are also sensitive to food colorings and additives in processed foods, because these chemicals are phenols, which slow down SULT pathways even more. Without knowing it, people are literally clogging their SULT pathway with toxins, oxalates, food colorings, and more. As discussed earlier, because of the action of the Sat1 transporter, when oxalate levels go up, sulfate levels go down.

As if losing sulfate wasn't bad enough, high oxalates also cause the body to lose vitamin B6. B vitamins are so important for our health: they activate our genetic pathways, produce energy, enhance detoxification, and enable our cells to survive. Vitamin B6, aka pyridoxine, is a particularly important B vitamin. It has many roles in the body, particularly in the liver, where it helps to transform amino acids to promote growth, repair, and detoxification. Fortunately, this isn't a biochemistry textbook and I won't bore you with all the intricate details of how B6 is used in our bodies. What I will highlight is how B6 is very useful in helping people with high oxalates and hyperoxaluria.

In a 2011 study with individuals with a genetic type of high oxalates called primary hyperoxaluria type 1, researchers discovered that about 30 percent of individuals with this genetic disease experienced a reversal of their condition when they took supplements of vitamin B6.[19] That surprising result is confirmed by another study that was published more than 20 years prior. In this earlier study, researchers concluded that taking vitamin B6 in high, therapeutic dosages of 5mg per kg per day was effective at reducing a high level of urinary oxalates.[20] The patients taking elevated doses of B6 (up to 400 mg/day in some individuals) for 18 months reported no side effects from the B vitamin therapy. (How many pharmaceutical drugs can say that?) These studies lend credence to the idea of how safe and effective vitamin B6 can be in people with oxalate toxicity.

At first glance, it might seem that 5mg per kg per day of a vitamin like B6 is too high a dose, but there is sound physiologic science behind this idea. As shown in Figure 5.4, the liver enzyme AGT is responsible for converting glyoxylate, the precursor molecule to oxalates, into the much-needed amino acid glycine.[21] Thus, the faster the AGT enzyme is functioning, the more rapidly the liver can convert glyoxylate into glycine, preventing the production of oxalates. And because AGT requires B6 to function, we can see how therapeutic B6 levels may be needed to increase the speed and function of AGT, leading to fewer oxalate molecules being formed. Whenever there are elevated levels of oxalates due to a genetic, digestive, or metabolic problem, B6 should be considered a useful and effective means to help detoxify this molecule from the body.

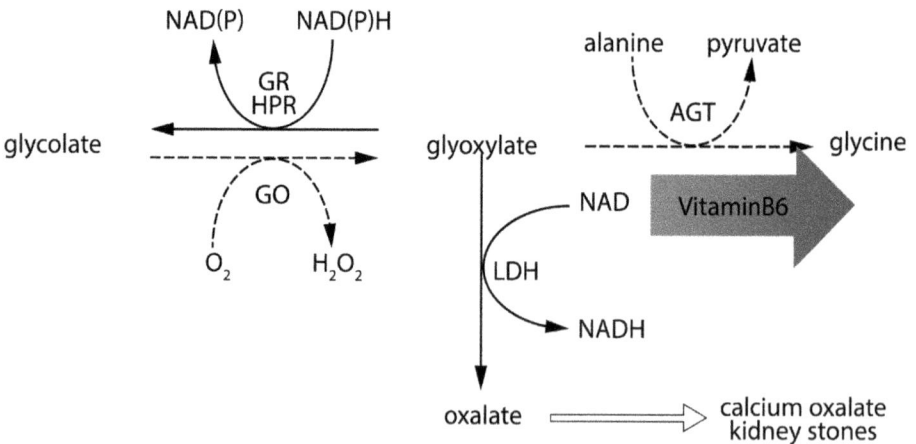

Figure 5.4 - *Pathway for oxalate removal and detoxification*

THE LOW SULFATE, HIGH OXALATE PHENOTYPE

Now that you have seen how oxalates can impact our B6 levels, let's turn our attention again to the all-important sulfate molecule. By taking a closer look at the oxalate-sulfate connection, we can identify the widespread methylation and biochemical problems caused by high oxalates. By finding the relationships among oxalates, sulfates, kidney health, hormones, liver detoxification, and more, we can recognize the high oxalate, low sulfate phenotype.

The big idea with oxalate toxicity is it causes problems in the liver and kidney—our two most important organs of detoxification. Although high oxalates will cause liver problems and a loss of B6, it is in the kidney where the oxalate causes us to lose much of our precious sulfate. The kidney is a critical player with any sulfate problem because the organ is responsible for keeping our sulfate levels in balance.[22] The kidney must swap a molecule of oxalate for a molecule of sulfate through the Sat1 transporter, and when oxalates are high, a loss of sulfate into the urine results. Urine sulfate levels have been a confusing subject for many patients, researchers, and doctors who study methylation and genetic pathways. Everyone wants to know where this sulfate is coming from, and I believe the answer has to do with oxalates and kidney polymorphisms.

Many people have used urine sulfate test strips and found high sulfate levels of greater than 1200-1600 mg/L. This has caused a lot of confusion, because very few people know why this happens. Online message boards and chat rooms are filled with pages of perplexing urine sulfate information. Some people say it's bad to have high urine sulfates; some say it's good, because it means the body is getting enough and eliminating the extra. The advice ranges from the practical to the absurd, with many deciding to avoid sulfur because of a high urine sulfate reading. But since sulfur and sulfate are essential for our health and well-being, I am not convinced that avoiding sulfur based on a urine sulfate test is valid—in fact, it's probably the worst thing you can do!

Remember from earlier that the most common reason for high oxalates is some kind of chronic gallbladder and gut problem. But not everyone has oxalate, gallbladder, or gut issues, yet high amounts of sulfate are being dumped into their urine. In these cases, the loss of sulfur must be coming from some other problem, and a genetic issue would make the most sense. Similar to our methylation cycle, where the MTHFR gene SNPs slow down the activation of folate, research now shows people with certain genes are prone to wasting their sulfate into the urine.

Cutting-edge research has identified that some people have a polymorphism in the NaS1 transporter found in the kidney, the main enzyme for balancing our sulfate levels. Although the science is still a bit murky on this, studies have identified two polymorphisms in the kidney that predispose us to losing sulfate. The NaS1 transporter SNPs were shown to reduce sulfate transport by an incredible 60 to 100 percent.[23] This means that for individuals with these NaS1 polymorphisms, a massive amount of sulfur is being lost in the urine on a daily basis. If someone with a NaS1 +/+ polymorphism also develops an oxalate problem, then look out, because we can expect them to have dangerously low sulfate levels. And you are about to learn how low sulfate levels make us really, really sick!

Could this NaS1 SNP be a major reason why many people are seeing a drastic loss of sulfate into their urine? I certainly think so! And if these individuals with NaS1 polymorphisms see high sulfates in their urine, and then decide to go "low sulfur," can you imagine the problems that will result?

Current biochemical research has been providing us with powerful studies that show what can happen to our bodies when oxalates rise and sulfate levels plummet. To figure out what happens when sulfate is lost in the urine, researchers developed a mouse model that was born without the NaS1 transporter. Researchers basically created a mouse that mimics people who are born with the NaS1 polymorphisms—that is, these mice were born without the ability to absorb sulfate in the kidney, and they developed severe sulfate deficiencies. Many of the health problems these low-sulfate, high-oxalate phenotype mice developed will sound familiar:

- Stunted growth

- Slow metabolism

- Altered behavior

- Decreased insulin function

- Elevated LDL and total cholesterol

- Increased liver stress and fatty liver deposits

- Impaired detoxification and upregulated SULT genes

- Low cortisol, DHEA, and adrenal hormone deficiency

- Increased colitis and inflammatory bowel disease

- Decreased mucus production in the gut

- Increased gut permeability (leaky gut)

- Susceptibility to aggressive gut bacteria

- Reduced metallothionein expression and heavy-metal detoxification

- Increased size and vascularity of tumors

- Excess serotonin in the blood and decreased serotonin in the brain

- Autism linked to sulfate wasting

LOW SULFATE LIVER PROBLEMS

The liver is the main organ for detoxification. This genius organ performs thousands of tasks every second we are alive. We often take what the liver does for granted, because it is so efficient at keeping our body in balance. But if high oxalates or genetic SNPs cause us to lose sulfate in the urine, the liver will take a big hit.

To understand just how serious low sulfate can be for the liver, consider the recent study of mice that are born without the NaS1 transporter.

Researchers bred mice that suffered from chronic urine sulfate loss and then looked at how sulfate loss impacted the animals' growth, detoxification, and methylation-related pathways. The results are quite alarming. Mice lacking the NaS1 transporter suffered from decreased growth, decreased serum insulin-like growth factor I (IGF-I) levels, altered serum bile acid concentrations, elevated LDL and total cholesterol, fatty livers, increase of SULT detox genes, and enlarged livers.[24] In addition to those major liver stressors, these mice also showed a 71 percent decrease in metallothionein expression. What this means is that the body doesn't just lose liver function with low sulfate; it also loses a key part of the methylation cycle. Without metallothionein, the body cannot defend itself against toxic heavy metals and is susceptible to neurotoxicity and brain inflammation.[25, 26] And as we all know, people with chronic disease need all the help with detoxification and inflammation they can get.

SULFATE LOSS AND HORMONES

When sulfate levels are low, the body won't just have disturbed liver function, but it will also suffer with all kinds of hormone problems, because the body uses sulfate molecules to inactivate hormones. In a 2008 study also using NaS1-deficient mice, researchers showed that blood levels were reduced 50 percent for cortisol, 30 percent for DHEA, and 40 percent for DHEA-S compared to non-deficient mice.[27] This massive loss of blood hormones was accompanied by a 1500 percent increase of cortisol spilt into the urine and lost as well. Of course, losing all this cortisol from the blood and the urine will greatly stress the body's nutritional and adrenal reserves. It takes a lot of energy and nutritional resources to build a hormone from scratch. And anyone who has suffered with adrenal fatigue can tell you that when the body is tired and run down, it doesn't do a very good job of building hormones. We know that hormone production requires energy, vitamins, minerals, and essential fatty acids—things people with chronic health issues have in short supply.

Consider how the body's hormonal needs are always changing. We need different hormones at night than during the day and different hormones during rest and play, and women who are menstruating need different levels of hormones throughout the month. Suffice it to say our hormonal needs are always fluctuating through our days, months, and years of life. Luckily, the body has developed a smart method for balancing our hormone levels: it sulfates them. Rather than spending energy removing a hormone only to have to build another one to replace it, the body inactivates steroid hormones by attaching a sulfate molecule.

In fact, many of the hormones we test for in clinical practice such as progesterone, estrogen, cortisol, and DHEA are stored in the blood in a sulfated form. And clinicians often order tests for DHEA-S, Progesteron-S, and others to look at the blood levels of the sulfated hormones and provide a more detailed picture of the hormone levels in the body. The body uses sulfate molecules to keep the hormones in circulation and to store them until later when the body needs to reactivate them. In this way, the body is more efficient, because it can activate and inactivate a hormone simply by removing a molecule of sulfate. This takes much less effort than building a hormone from scratch every time. So when sulfate levels are low or nonexistent, there is a severe drop in hormones and greater stress placed on the adrenals and sex organs to compensate.

LOW SULFATE AND GUT PROBLEMS

Now that we've looked at how high oxalates and low sulfate disrupt health, I wish I could end the discussion here. But if I did, I wouldn't be giving you the whole story, including how the loss of sulfate drastically impacts gut health. Now that you have seen how low sulfate creates liver and hormone problems, let's consider another critical part of our health. Gut health is the foundation for the health of every other system in our body. And the balance of our gut microbes determines in large part the health of our gut. We simply cannot have a healthy digestive system if we cannot sustain and maintain healthy bacteria in our colon and small intestine.

The gut is a very big place. If we were to unwrap and spread out our gut from the esophagus to the rectum, it would cover about 350 square feet, roughly half the size of a badminton court. That means there's a huge surface area packed and folded into our abdominal area. This great surface area helps us to absorb nutrients better and provides space for tens of trillions of microorganisms to live within us.

Just like bugs and insects in the forest need a place to live and food to eat, so, too, do the gut bugs in our bowels. To provide our gut bacteria with a sustainable living condition, the cells that line our gut produce mucus. This mucus coats and protects our own cells while also providing food and shelter for the bacteria we depend on for survival. And since we cannot make mucus without sulfate, any low sulfate problem will create a gut issue.

Current research highlights how problematic low sulfate is for our digestive system. In a study published in 2009, researchers discovered that low-sulfate mice suffered with inflammatory bowel disease, decreased mucus production, leaky gut, and aggressive bacterial infections.[28] Another study published in 2014 confirms that low sulfate, in addition to slowing growth and liver function, has a major negative impact on gut function.[29]

The important take-away here is that once the body loses sulfate, mucus production in the gut is interrupted. Since our good, healthy probiotics depend on the mucus for survival, any loss of mucus production will lead to a loss of healthy probiotics. Without a healthy mucous layer, the cells that line our gut will be unable to defend themselves against toxins, while aggressive bacteria will injure and inflame the lining of our gut. Keep in mind that sulfate is required to build strong molecular bonds, such as the bonds in our skin, cartilage, bones, and other connective tissues. It is also required to make mucous be sticky and coat the lining of the bowel. If the body is depleted of sulfate, either because of a kidney polymorphism or an oxalate toxicity, mucous production and gut health is going to suffer.

LOW SULFATES, CANCER, AND AUTISM

Two more pieces to this oxalate-sulfate puzzle must be shared. As if it wasn't enough that low sulfate seriously hampers our liver, hormones, and gut function, studies also show that low sulfate impacts serotonin levels, cancer growth, and autism spectrum disorders. We all know that cancer, depression, and developmental disorders such as autism spectrum disorders are now epidemic in our society, but few people realize how low sulfate can make these problems worse.

To understand how low sulfate impacts cancer, researchers looked again at the NaS1 -/- low-sulfate mouse model. The researchers studied how very low sulfate levels can affect tumor growth, and the results were astounding. In a study published in 2010, researchers discovered that tumors grew 12 times faster and had more than double the blood vessels in the low-sulfate mice versus the normal-sulfate mice.[30] When mice have cancer and low sulfate levels at the same time, the cancer thrives in that environment and becomes much more aggressive. This suggests a critical role for sulfate to play in keeping our bodies healthy, and it shows that low sulfate levels make it that much more difficult for the body to overcome a chronic disease like cancer. We humans aren't as simple a creature as a mouse, but we share a lot of the same biochemistry. Isn't it possible that we may also suffer more aggressive cancer if our sulfate levels drop? The evidence suggests this is a real possibility.

When researchers turned their attention to low sulfate and serotonin, they found that neurotransmitters are also greatly impacted by sulfate issues. Researchers in 2007 used low-sulfate mice and found that blood serotonin levels doubled while brain serotonin levels were reduced by about 12 percent compared to normal mice.[31] At first, a study like this may not sound very important, but let's break down what these scientists are saying: When sulfate is lost in the urine (as happens with high oxalates), there is less sulfate available to help us balance neurotransmitters. Sulfate is glued to neurotransmitters and hormones such as serotonin, progesterone, estrogen, etc., as a way to regulate them. Sulfate allows the body to produce these molecules but keeps them in an inactivated state to use when the body needs them in the future. Like a farmer who grows extra food and stores it for use in the winter, the body stores sulfate reserves to use when it needs it to regulate our hormones.

Can you imagine how challenging it would be for your body to live without sulfate and the ability to inactivate your hormones and neurotransmitters? What a mess! Since these mice lacked the ability to regulate their serotonin, they ended up with way too much of it floating around in their bodies. It might seem like a good thing to have higher serotonin, but when we look at the bigger picture and realize that our body also uses sulfate to regulate many other hormones, we can see a potential disaster here. Without sufficient sulfate in our bodies, we not only lose control of neurotransmitters, but we also cannot balance our other critical hormones that keep us healthy. And given how many people are suffering with adrenal fatigue, infertility, menopause, andropause (male menopause), and other hormone issues, it's obvious that low sulfate is a much bigger problem than most of us think.

The research on sulfate is amazing partly because of how many different conditions are related to it. And this is especially true of the autism epidemic, where sulfate is critical for children with ASD concerns. Remember that in order for our body's detoxification system to work correctly, we need sulfate molecules available (technically, we need the PAPS molecule, a close derivative of sulfate). Our liver takes sulfate molecules, which are produced in the methylation cycle, and glues them to stuff we need to get rid of. The body glues sulfate to drugs, hormones, toxins, heavy metals, and other garbage that we must eliminate in order to be healthy. And you don't have to be a doctor or a researcher to know that children with autism have a problem with detoxification, and this means they have a problem with sulfate. Anything that lowers the availability of sulfate for their body to use is going to be a problem for autistic children. And that is precisely why high oxalates and low sulfate levels are especially harmful for these kids.

Although the cause of autism remains uncertain, the latest data from the Centers for Disease Control (CDC) shows that rates of autism continue to skyrocket. In 2000, rates of autism were 1 in 150, but by the year 2010, autism affected 1 in 68, with boys affected four times more often than girls, at a rate of 1 in 48 boys versus only 1 in 189 girls.[32] If the CDC's own data wasn't enough of a shocker, we have some cutting-edge PhD research that paints an even darker picture.

According to Dr. Stephanie Seneff, a research scientist at Massachusetts Institute of Technology (MIT), by 2032, we can expect to see 50 percent of all children affected by autism. This number might sound preposterous, but Dr. Seneff is a mathematics expert and bases her calculations on the current rate of increase. In other words, if we don't change the rate at which ASD issues are occurring, her numbers will prove true in less than two decades!

Another important aspect of Dr. Seneff's research relates to the increasing ASD rates and the use of genetically modified food sprayed with the toxin glyphosate. She has highlighted the connection between genetically modified foods and the poisons used to grow them compared to the rates of ASD.[33] I will admit that correlation is not causation, so more studies are needed to confirm this. But at the same time, there is a clear relationship between use of glyphosate and increasing rates of autism disorders, as shown in Figure 5.5. I would recommend that we not eat GMO foods while we wait years for more studies to prove the toxicity of these genetically modified "foods"!

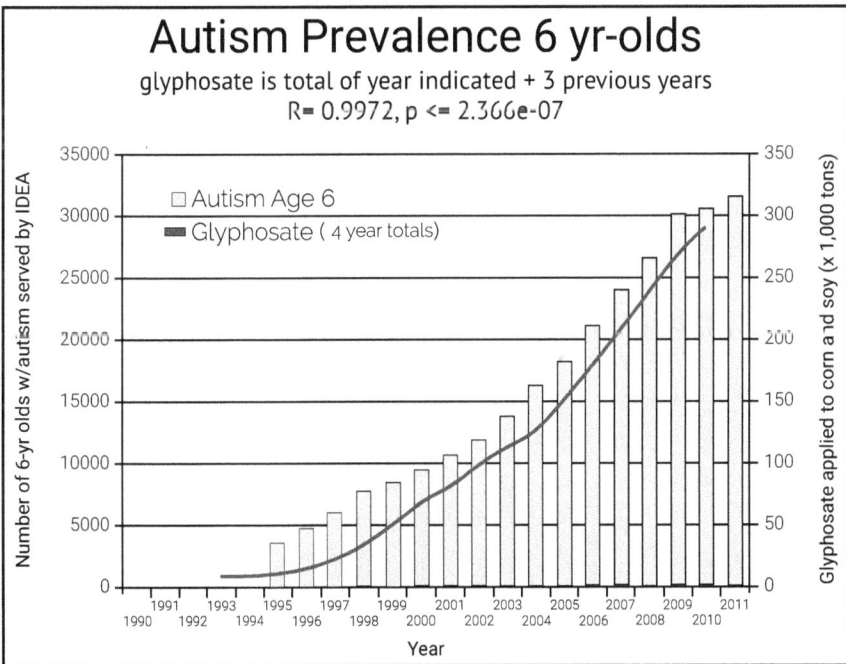

Figure 5.5 - *2013 research study showing 99 percent correlation between use of glyphosate and rise in autism spectrum disorders in the United States.[34] (Used with permission)*

Here's one final study to share with you on oxalates: Researchers looked for a connection between autistic individuals and urine sulfate levels. In a study published in 2013, researchers investigated autistic children to determine whether they had NaS1 SNPs and to measure how much sulfate they lost in their urine. They found that 78 percent of autistic children have NaS1 kidney polymorphisms and that 60 percent of these autistic children with this polymorphism end up wasting high amounts of sulfate into their urine.[35] This confirms that autistic children are prone to low sulfate levels. This study alone may not carry a ton of weight, but when we consider the impact that low sulfate can have on our bodies, we can see the potential.

I've discussed how low sulfate leads to changes in growth, behavior, gut function, immune health, and slower detoxification. Clearly these health issues are familiar problems for individuals struggling with ASD. I want to clarify that I am not saying that low sulfate is the cause of autism. However, given how important sulfate is for the health of our cells, it's obvious that anything that lowers sulfate levels will put stress on our bodies. Because those with autism already face many hurdles, any additional biochemical stresses on these individuals should be avoided at all costs. This is why it is so important to look at oxalate and sulfate issues with all patients who are dealing with chronic health concerns such as ASD and developmental issues.

CONCLUSION

As I close this chapter, I want to reiterate that oxalates are an important part of the chronic disease puzzle. Because oxalates injure our kidneys and reduce the function of our liver, we need to be aware of oxalates in our diets and bodies. This is especially true in individuals who are living with serious methylation problems. People who don't methylate well already have a susceptibility to stress, toxins, and gut problems. Adding an oxalate problem on top of that just creates another, often unrecognized, hurdle for the body to overcome.

Despite the potential toxicity of oxalates and the fact they are found in much of our food, our bodies are well equipped to deal with this foodborne toxin. The mechanism the body uses to prevent oxalate problems is very simple: it requires a healthy gallbladder and gut. This is why we always, always, make sure the gut is functioning as we begin to help patients heal. But since gut health is usually ignored and not understood in traditional healthcare systems, we will likely see more oxalate issues creating chronic health problems. In my practice, we address oxalate problems right away, and you can, too, by following the genius body advice in the following protocol.

OXALATE PROTOCOL

In the beginning of the healing process, people with oxalate issues should be cautious and lower their oxalate intake slowly. Many patients have reported experiencing an oxalate "dumping" syndrome if they go from high oxalates to low too quickly. The best advice is to lower your oxalate intake by 5 to 10 percent each week until you settle into a mild oxalate diet. It isn't necessary to be strictly 100 percent low oxalate for most people; just reducing slowly from high to medium/moderate plus proper supplementation seems to be the right protocol for most. After that initial period, individuals with a history of high oxalates may eat high-oxalate foods as long as they support their gut with calcium-citrate and bile support. I've provided information about which supplements are useful to help protect your body from oxalates. This is useful whether you are recovering from high oxalates or are just seeking to prevent them from becoming an issue in the future. You will find a list of websites with useful high oxalate food lists in appendix D.

RECOMMENDED LAB TESTING:

I recommend the Routine Blood Tests, Sulfite Urine Test, and the Organic Acid Test in appendix B for assessing the full extent of oxalate issues and vitamin deficiencies associated with high oxalates. To make full use of the information in this book, I recommend following the instructions found in appendix A to get your own detailed genetic report.

HIGH OXALATE PROTOCOL:

<u>Bone Support Vegetarian</u> – 2 capsules at the beginning of each meal. Provides gut-specific calcium-citrate, which binds up excess oxalates in the diet, preventing oxalate toxicity in the liver, kidney, and rest of the tissues. When treating high oxalates, take this product with every single meal. Once oxalate levels lower and become balanced, this product should be taken with high oxalate meals such as smoothies, kale and spinach salads, etc.† (Nutridyn)

<u>Stress Essentials Relax</u> – 2 capsules 3 times per day with meals. Helps to support glutathione production in the liver and provides high doses of taurine to improve bile flow; also provides B6, which is necessary for oxalate detoxification inside the liver.† (Nutridyn)

<u>Sulforaphane Complex</u> – 1 or 2 capsules 2 times per day with meals. Provides a high-potency source of sulfate from broccoli sprouts, which helps improve sulfation and antioxidant production.† (Nutridyn)

<u>UltraBiotic Daily Multi-Strain</u> – 1 capsules 2 times per day. Provides the *L. plantarum* strain to help break down oxalates in the intestines.†(Nutridyn)

<u>Vitamin B6</u> – 1 capsule 1 or 2 times per day. Additional B6 support for individuals with high oxalate levels.† (Nutridyn)

<u>L-Lysine</u> – 2 capsules 1 to 3 times per day. Provides amino acid lysine, which is necessary for our bodies to be able to utilize the B6 molecule.

---

†This statement has not been evaluated by the FDA. This product is not intended to diagnose, treat, cure, or prevent any disease. The information provided in this book is intended for your general knowledge only and is not a substitute for professional medical advice or treatment for specific medical conditions. You should not use this information to diagnose or treat a health problem or disease without consulting with a qualified healthcare provider. Please consult your healthcare provider with any questions or concerns you may have regarding your condition. Never disregard professional medical advice or delay in seeking it because of something you have read in this book.

Many people with chronic virus infections, cold sores, herpes, low B6 function, and oxalate issues are low in lysine.† (Nutridyn)

Because oxalates are not a well-recognized health problem, getting good advice about this issue can be difficult. Not only that, but there is a great deal of conflicting evidence about what is the best diet for people with high oxalate issues. Although I have worked hard to explain the issue with oxalates in this chapter, you may be interested in more support in this area. For more insight and support on dealing with oxalates, visit the Facebook group Trying Low Oxalates. This group is run by Susan Owens, who is likely the most educated and experienced oxalate researcher and practitioner in the world. Many of my patients have found good advice and support through the Trying Low Oxalate group.

REFERENCES

1. Low Oxalate Diet May Help Prevent Kidney Stones. University of Pittsburgh Medical Center website. www.upmc.com/patients-visitors/education/nutrition/pages/low-oxalate-diet.aspx. Accessed October 17, 2015.

2. Nguyen, Q.V., A. Kälin, U. Drouve, et al. Sensitivity to meat protein intake and hyperoxaluria in idiopathic calcium stone formers. *Kidney Int.* (2001) 59(6): 2273-81.

3. Kumar R., J.C. Lieske, M.L. Collazo-Clavell, et al. Fat malabsorption and increased intestinal oxalate absorption are common after Roux-en-Y gastric bypass surgery. *Surgery.* (2011) 149(5): 654-61.

4. Common Surgical Procedures. The University of Chicago Medicine website. www.uchospitals.edu/online-library/content=P01392. Accessed November 27, 2015.

5. Marengo, S.R., A.M. Romani. Oxalate in renal stone disease: the terminal metabolite that just won't go away. *Nat Clin Pract Nephrol.* (2008) 4(7): 368-77.

6. Yiu, A.J., D. Callaghan, R. Sultana, et al. Vascular Calcification and Stone Disease: A New Look towards the Mechanism. *J Cardiovasc Dev Dis.* (2015) 2(3): 141-64.

7. Dobbins, J.W., H.J. Binder. Importance of the colon in enteric hyperoxaluria. *N Engl J Med.* (1977) 296(6): 298-301.

8. Evan, A.P. Physiopathology and etiology of stone formation in the kidney and the urinary tract. *Pediatr Nephrol.* (2010) 25(5): 831-41.

9. Shaw, W. Oxalates Control is a Major New Factor in Autism Therapy. Great Plains Laboratory website. www.greatplainslaboratory.com/home/eng/oxalates.asp. Accessed November 27, 2015.

10. Ghio, A.J., V.L. Roggli, T.P. Kennedy, et al. Calcium oxalate and iron accumulation in sarcoidosis. *Sarcoidosis Vasc Diffuse Lung Dis.* (2000) 17(2): 140-50.

11. Ott, S.M., D.L. Andress, D.J. Sherrard. Bone oxalate in a long-term hemodialysis patient who ingested high doses of vitamin C. *Am J Kidney Dis.* (1986) 8(6): 450-54.

12. Hall, B.M., J.C. Walsh, J.S. Horvath, et al. Peripheral neuropathy complicating primary hyperoxaluria. *J Neurol Sci.* (1976) 29(2-4): 343-49.

13. Sahin, G., M.F. Acikalin, A.U. Yalcin. Erythropoietin resistance as a result of oxalosis in bone marrow. *Clin Nephrol.* (2005) 63(5): 402-4.

14. Hess, B., C. Jost, L. Zipperle, et al. High-calcium intake abolishes hyperoxaluria and reduces urinary crystallization during a 20-fold normal oxalate load in humans. *Nephrol Dial Transplant.* (1998) 13(9): 2241-47.

15. Berg, C. Alkaline citrate in prevention of recurrent calcium oxalate stones. *Scand J Urol Nephrol*

Suppl. (1990) 130: 1-83.

16. Ohana, E., N. Shcheynikov, O.W. Moe, et al. SLC26A6 and NaDC-1 transporters interact to regulate oxalate and citrate homeostasis. *J Am Soc Nephrol.* (2013) 24(10): 1617–26.

17. Ostojic, S.M., ed. *Steroids–From Physiology to Clinical Medicine.* 1st ed. InTech, November 21, 2012 under CC BY 3.0 license. Accessed June 12, 2015.

18. SLC26A1–Sulfate anion transporter 1. Uniprot.org website. www.uniprot.org/uniprot/Q9H2B4. Accessed October 27, 2015.

19. Robijn, S., B. Hoppe, B.A. Vervaet, et al. Hyperoxaluria: a gut-kidney axis? *Kidney Int.* (2011) 80(11): 1146–58.

20. Mitwalli, A., A. Ayiomamitis, L. Grass, et al. Control of hyperoxaluria with large doses of pyridoxine in patients with kidney stones. *Int Urol Nephrol.* (1988) 20(4): 353-59.

21. Behnam, J.T., E.L. Williams, S. Brink, et al. Reconstruction of human hepatocyte glyoxylate metabolic pathways in stably transformed Chinese-hamster ovary cells. *Biochem J.* (2006) 394(Pt 2): 409-16.

22. Markovich, D. Physiological roles of renal anion transporters NaS1 and Sat1. *Am J Physiol Renal Physiol.* (2011) 300(6): F1267-70.

23. Lee, S., P.A. Dawson, A.K. Hewavitharana, et al. Disruption of NaS1 sulfate transport function in mice leads to enhanced acetaminophen-induced hepatotoxicity. *Hepatology.* (2006) 43(6): 1241-47.

24. Dawson, P.A., B. Gardiner, S. Grimmond, et al. Transcriptional profile reveals altered hepatic lipid and cholesterol metabolism in hyposulfatemic NaS1 null mice. *Physiol Genomics.* (2006) 26(2): 116-24.

25. Stankovic, R.K., R.S. Chung, M. Penkowa. Metallothioneins I and II: neuroprotective significance during CNS pathology. *Int J Biochem Cell Biol.* (2007) 39(3): 484-89.

26. Yu, X., J. Guo, H. Fang, et al. Basal metallothionein-I/II protects against NMDA-mediated oxidative injury in cortical neuron/astrocyte cultures. *Toxicology.* (2011) 282(1-2): 16-22.

27. Dawson, P.A., B. Gardiner, S. Lee, et al. Kidney transcriptome reveals altered steroid homeostasis in NaS1 sulfate transporter null mice. *J Steroid Biochem Mol Biol.* (2008) 112(1-3): 55-62.

28. Dawson, P.A., S. Huxley, B. Gardiner, et al. Reduced mucin sulfonation and impaired intestinal barrier function in the hyposulfataemic NaS1 null mouse. *Gut.* (2009) 58(7): 910-19.

29. Markovich, D. Na+-sulfate cotransporter SLC13A1. *Pflugers Arch.* (2014) 466(1): 131-37.

30. Dawson, P.A., A. Choyce, C. Chuang, et al. Enhanced tumor growth in the NaS1 sulfate transporter null mouse. *Cancer Sci.* (2010) 101(2): 369-73.

31. Lee, S., J.P. Kesby, M.D. Muslim, et al. Hyperserotonaemia and reduced brain serotonin levels in NaS1 sulphate transporter null mice. *Neuroreport.* (2007) 18(18): 1981-85.

32. Baio, J. Prevalence of Autism Spectrum Disorder Among Children Aged 8 Years—Autism and Developmental Disabilities Monitoring Network, 11 Sites, United States. (2010) *Surveillance Summaries.* (March 28, 2014) 63(SS02): 1-21.

33. Samsel A., S. Seneff. Glyphosate, pathways to modern diseases III: Manganese, neurological diseases, and associated pathologies. *Surgical Neurology International.* (2015) 6: 45.

34. Ibid.

35. Bowling, F.G., H.S. Heussler, A. McWhinney, et al. Plasma and urinary sulfate determination in a cohort with autism. *Biochem Genet.* (2013) 51(1-2): 147-53.

6.

MTHFR AND SIBO: WHEN TOO MUCH OF A GOOD THING IS A BAD THING

Never go to excess, but let moderation be your guide.

—Marcus Tullius Cicero

As I mentioned, before you treat your methylation problem or other health problems, you must first heal the gut. If you aren't convinced yet, I will show you again why this idea is so important. This chapter will highlight a growing gut problem in our society called *small intestine bacterial overgrowth,* or SIBO. As you will see, SIBO is caused by several major issues that plague us, including poor nutrition and diet choices, excess stress, chemical toxicity, and excessive dependence on pharmaceutical drugs. Combine all that with less-than-optimum methylation genetics and you get a recipe for disaster. Unfortunately, our collective overuse of antibiotics is a big part of this problem. To support that concept, I will show you studies that highlight how the standard of care in our medical system is destroying our digestive tracts.

But first, it's important to recognize that the health of the gut determines the health of the body. This is a well-known fact. The latest research estimates that the adult human body contains around 4 trillion cells—at first blush that might sound like a lot.[1] Consider, however, that we each carry around anywhere from 2 to 6 pounds of bugs on and in our bodies, which means we have at least 10 times the number of cells of microorganisms (mostly bacteria, but also some other types of critters) than we do our own cells.[2] Suddenly, those 4 trillion cells don't seem as many compared to the 40 trillion living in our gut and on our bodies! This mass of bacteria lives in harmony with us most of the time and helps make sure our immune system is functioning and we are able to digest our food. Without these bacteria in our gut and on our skin, we cannot experience lasting health and well-being.

But what happens when these bacteria and bugs become imbalanced? What are the implications to our health when we have an overgrowth of bacteria in the gut as occurs in SIBO? When the small intestine is over-whelmed with bacteria, it can have major impacts on our methylation cycle. Living with an excess of bacteria in your small intestine can make methylation problems much worse.

THE SIBO PROBLEM

SIBO is like an infection made up of noninfectious bacteria. A SIBO prob-lem is different from getting food poisoning or dealing with a dangerous strain of *Clostridium difficile* or *Salmonella enterica*. It's not an infection in the traditional sense. Instead, SIBO is an overgrowth of bacteria that is nor-mally found in our digestive tract. As you can see in Figure 6.1, SIBO occurs when the gut bacteria normally found in the colon and ileum grow wildly and end up near the top of the small intestine. Bacteria that are nonpatho-genic, healthy types are very good at pooping out vitamins for our body to use. Though a moderate, balanced amount of healthy bacteria supports optimum health, too much of this bacteria can become a bad thing.

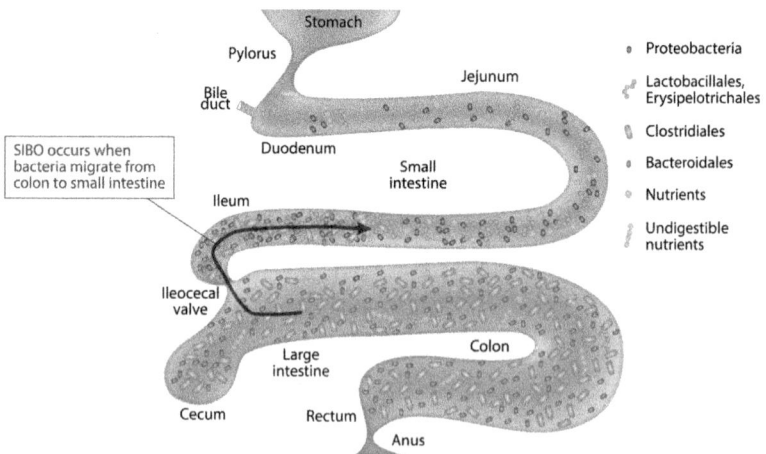

Figure 6.1 - *Migration of bacteria from the colon and ileum into the upper small intestine*

The SIBO problem is a double-edged sword. On one side are the excess bacteria in the small intestine, which interfere with the process of digestion. Just like people, pets, and plants, bacteria need to eat in order to survive. So when the bacteria populations explode in the small intestine, they also eat much more than normal. If the bacteria are eating too much of the food we consume, there is less food and nutrition available for our body. This is why malabsorption is so common with SIBO problems.

On the other side of the SIBO sword is the fact that these bacterial populations actively poop out vitamins that our bodies absorb. Clearly, this is advantageous in a balanced and healthy gut. But when bacteria levels go through the roof, they can actually excrete too much of one vitamin, blocking the absorption of another. We see this relationship in SIBO all the time, as patients experience elevated levels of certain B vitamins such as folic acid along with low levels of B12, vitamin D, iron, and others. This is a problem because the bacteria down there can produce folic acid while simultaneously causing all kinds of other digestive issues.

THE FOLIC ACID PROBLEM

There is a controversy surrounding folic acid, a synthetic B vitamin hat was created in a laboratory in 1946.[3] Many assume that folic acid is a fake, man-made vitamin that came into existence only after we synthesized it. But that isn't the case. New research shows that the bacteria involved with SIBO actually excrete large amounts of folic acid, and we absorb that folic acid into our bodies.

The truth is, our bodies have been exposed to folic acid for a very, very long time. Even if we don't eat processed foods fortified with folic acid or take supplements containing the same, our gut bugs have the ability to make folic acid by themselves. In fact, research proves that several different species of *Bifidobacterium* bacteria commonly found in our small intestine are capable of producing folic acid.[4, 5, 6, 7] This is why having too much bacteria in our gut can lead to too much folic acid being released and absorbed into our bodies. When someone has SIBO, or an overgrowth of "good" *Bifidobacterium* bacteria in the small intestine, the bacteria can produce excess amounts of folic acid. In fact, one of the main diagnostic criteria for SIBO is a high level of unmetabolized folic acid (UMFA) present in the bloodstream.[8]

Although it is clear that folic acid is a natural substance found in nature, excess folic acid is not something we want building up inside our bodies. Folic acid in high amounts can be toxic to our cells, especially cells in the liver and brain. Whether the folic acid comes from supplements or fortified foods, as most people assume, or if it comes from a SIBO-style gut problem is irrelevant. The fact is that folic acid in high amounts in people with methylation genetics is a problem. It can lead to high blood levels of unmetabolized folic acid, which as Dr. Lynch and other researchers have shown, can impair the methylation cycle in people with MTHFR genes.[9]

The key to understand here is that many patients are suffering because their bodies are full of folic acid and they don't have enough activated folate inside their cells—a real methylation problem. Supporting this concept, research has demonstrated that folic acid is able to starve the cell of needed *activated* folate (L 5-methyltetrahydrofolate), weakening the methylation cycle.[10] Although there is still a lingering debate about this issue in the scientific literature, it is clear that having too much folic acid can impair the methylation cycle. Here is how it works:

1. Folic acid comes from fortified food, supplements, and gut bacteria. Every person on Earth gets some folic acid into their bodies from the action of our gut bacteria. We get in trouble when the bacteria in our colon grows and moves into the small intestine. Normally, only a small number of bacteria is found in the small intestine, but when the digestive system becomes imbalanced, the population of bacteria in the small intestine can increase, creating a condition of SIBO. Excess gut bacteria and poor dietary choices lead to a buildup of folic acid inside the body.

2. Folic acid and folate both enter the cell through the same receptor. If there is an excess of folic acid, it is harder for the activated folate to get into the cell. The more folic acid you have inside your bloodstream, the less often activated folate will get to the

receptor. In other words, there is competition between folic acid and folate, and when folic acid is elevated, it wins the competition to enter the cell.

3. In a person without methylation or MTHFR issues, this poses fewer problems, because folic acid is converted to folate in their methylation cycles at a normal rate. For those with methylation issues, excess folic acid makes it harder to create methyl donors. Since MTHFR is often slowed down along with MTR, MTRR, DHFR, and other SNPs, having high doses of folic acid can slow down the methylation cycle and create chronic disease.

This explains why folic acid in high amounts can make problems flare up for individuals with methylation issues, making them feel worse. People with methylation defects need more activated folate inside their cells, not less, so excess folic acid can worsen inherited methylation problems. And because SIBO infections continuously produce folic acid, many people with bad reactions to folic acid actually have a gut problem first and a methylation problem second. For individuals with untreated gut infections such as SIBO, taking more folate isn't wise until the gut is working better. Given the idea that folic acid may cause methylation issues, there is legitimate reason to be concerned about exposure to excess folic acid in foods and medications. We should always read labels to know what we are putting in our bodies or serving our families for dinner. However, we must keep in mind that another major cause of excess folic acid in the body is a raging gut infection!

Keep in mind that there are multiple reasons for SIBO infections to occur. As I will show later in this chapter, SIBO is caused by use of antibiotics, high-fat and high-carb junk food diets, proton-pump inhibitor (PPI) and acid-blocking drugs, and ileocecal valve dysfunction. Each of these triggers makes it easier for the bacteria that normally live in the colon to make their way up into the small intestine where they don't belong. In fact, people who have been on long-term antibiotics and/or PPIs often have the most challenging methylation issues. The reason is that those drugs—antibiotics and acid reflux medication—make it much more likely that an individual will suffer from SIBO-type problems. And with SIBO issues, we often see excess folic acid, low B12, and a host of other malnutrition/methylation issues that slow down the body's pathways and leave us feeling unwell. Truly a mess!

SNPS of Concern

Reacting negatively to B vitamins is a dead giveaway that someone has a SIBO gut infection. Bacteria poop out B vitamins too, and studies show that folic acid levels are way too high in people with SIBO. This high amount of folic acid irritates the methylation cycle, leading to increased levels of stress hormones with too much "fight-or-flight" responses. Not only that, but gut bugs also use B vitamins to grow and get more energy. When we have SIBO, all of our methylation SNPs are going to be feeling the pressure, and we can't optimize our genes until SIBO is treated.

The methylation cycle is very sensitive to the presence of SIBO in our gut. All of the genes we have mentioned so far including MTHFR, COMT, MAO, SULT, and ACE/AGT/ADD1 are impacted by SIBO. These SNPs create a tendency toward anxiety, insomnia, and elevated dopamine, adrenaline, and estrogen. When you add in a gut infection like SIBO, people suffer the most, because they become dopamine, adrenaline, and estrogen dominant all at the same time.

Following are some common health issues associated with SIBO: [11, 12]

- Low B12

- High folic acid

- Low iron

- Low vitamins A, D, E, and K

- Low Omega 3s and other fatty acids

- Difficulty gaining weight /failure to thrive

- Gas

- Diarrhea

- Bloating

- Abdominal pain

- Food in stool

- Fat in stool

- Acid reflux

- Malabsorption

- Difficulty losing weight / obesity

You don't need me to tell you that patients with methylation issues are often dealing with these symptoms every day. This further cements the idea that in order to heal the methylation cycle, we have to heal the gut. Remember that every supplement we take, every food we eat, and every beverage we drink interacts with the bacteria in our gut. If the gut is imbalanced and we have too much bacteria in the small intestine, we are going to have lukewarm results until we treat the gut problem. If we are suffering from a SIBO-style gut problem with health issues such as those listed, it will be very difficult to fix methylation issues until the gut is working better.

YOUR BEST FUT FORWARD

Sometimes genetic SNPs directly impact the balance of bacteria in the gut. The FUT2 polymorphism is a perfect example of this problem. The fucosyltransferase (FUT2) gene has a huge influence on how the cells that line our gut produce mucus. This mucus is critical for preventing leaky gut and contains compounds, oligosaccharides (a Greek word meaning "a few sugars"), which provide fuel for the good bacteria we depend on for health. Cutting-edge research has shown that individuals with FUT2 polymorphisms produce fewer oligosaccharides in the gut, which can lead to dysbiosis (a microbial unbalance or impairment) and increase the risk of Crohn's Disease.[13] Unfortunately, people with SIBO already have a bacterial problem; if FUT2 genes are present, the deck is truly stacked against them. Having FUT2 SNPs will make it more difficult for the healthy bugs to find food in the mucus layer of the gut, leading to a state in which the bad bugs outnumber the good ones.

On a related note, FUT2 has also been shown to influence how the gut develops in infants. When babies are breastfed by mothers carrying FUT2 SNPs, it takes longer for the good bugs to grow and become established in the gut. In 2015, researchers found that women with FUT2 genes produced less oligosaccharides in their breast milk, and the infants they fed took longer to grow a healthy population of *Bifidobacteria*.[14] Human milk oligosaccharides are used by *Bifidobacteria* as a fuel source, so when mothers with FUT2 genes produce breast milk, there is less food for the healthy *Bifidobacteria* to eat. Although a whole chapter could probably be devoted to this fascinating gene, just know that FUT2 increases the risk of gut inflammation and leaky gut as seen in SIBO. FUT2 polymorphisms represent another hidden weakness that can predispose us to gut problems. It is one more reason why we must take the high ground and work diligently to improve our digestion every day: our health literally hangs in the balance!

CONSIDERING SIBO CAUSES

Although it is very important to know what SIBO is, we still haven't answered the question of what actually causes SIBO. And if you are wondering how this problem occurs, you are really going to enjoy this section! We now know that SIBO can occur in the gut only when certain conditions are met—conditions that disrupt the normal function and chemistry of the digestive tract. In order for a gut infection like SIBO to take root, the environment in the intestines must be very out of balance. Although there are several distinct causes for a SIBO-style gut problem, not everyone with the risk factors will develop this problem, because the environment inside the digestive system is ultimately more important. Any successful treatment of SIBO must include measures to complement and enhance the natural digestive function and chemistry of the intestines. This is a critical piece that is missing from many popular SIBO protocols. As you will see, treating the environment isn't rocket science, but it does take a focused, concentrated effort.

When I meet a new patient and begin working with them to heal their methylation issues, the first thing we look at is their gastrointestinal health. Occasionally, a patient has experienced horrible, even dangerous, side effects of high dose methylation support. These individuals typically performed a genetic test with another doctor and discovered they have problems in their methylation pathways. These same patients are then put on 5, 10, or even 15 mg per day of methylfolate! In most cases, this causes a flare-up of their symptoms, including increased pain, tingling, numbness, headaches, anxiety, and insomnia. At worst, this kind of reckless approach can put people into the psychiatric ward. As you will come to see in this book, everything is connected—especially the gut and the methylation cycle. When there is a gut problem like SIBO, the body may not tolerate targeted methylation support, even when there is a genetic reason to do so. Said another way, it is very important to know if your gut is healthy before you begin working on methylation.

More than 3000 years ago, Hippocrates stated, "Let food be thy medicine and medicine be thy food." I am sure you will agree with me that this truism is as valid today as it was millennia ago. Unfortunately, the wisdom of using food as medicine is hijacked when the digestive system is harboring chronic infections and is simply unable to digest food correctly. If you don't have a properly functioning gut, then taking vitamins and eating healthy, nutritious food may not give you the benefit you were looking for; in fact, it may make you feel sick! Without a healthy gut, throwing vitamins and food into your body is like pouring fertilizer onto weeds. This is the number 1 reason why some people experience side effects and negative reactions from taking methylation support and other supplements.

To rule this problem out, I ask my patients many important questions:

- Have you ever taken any antibiotics? If so, how long ago and for how long did you take them?

- Have you ever taken steroid medications? If so, when and for how long?

- Have you had any issues with yeast or yeast infections?

- Have you ever been on birth control? If so, when and for how long?

- Do you have any constipation? Or diarrhea?

- Any history with acid reflux?

- Do you suffer from any abdominal pain? If so, is it above the belly button, or below? Right or left side?

- Do you see any undigested food in your stool?

- Can you tolerate fats in your diet? Even healthy ones like olive oil and fish oil?

- Do you have any gas, bloating, or discomfort following a meal?

- Any health issues or complications with
  your mother during pregnancy?

- Were you delivered vaginally or via C-section?

- Were you breast fed as an infant?

- Are you experiencing any unexplained weight loss?

- Do you get nauseated when you eat, or do you
  experience a loss of appetite due to food reactions?

It's not a stretch to say that many of you reading this book have at least one of these issues right now. The issues are everywhere in today's world. The reason these problems are so prevalent is that modern life is very hard on our digestive system. Despite the things our genius body does to help us digest our food, the many daily stressors we encounter cause our gut to take a beating. GI complaints continue to be a leading cause of doctor visits, and drugs that treat these issues are top sellers, grossing billions of dollars for the pharmaceutical industry.

With all this in mind, it may seem like we are destined to have SIBO and a dysfunctional gut no matter what. But don't let negativity get you down. The good news is that by understanding the three root causes of SIBO, we can not only heal our suffering, but we can also prevent SIBO from ever becoming a problem.

THE THREE ROOT CAUSES OF SIBO

Just because a person suffers from the symptoms associated with SIBO doesn't mean they actually have a SIBO problem. Many health problems share similar symptoms, so we want to acknowledge the symptoms but then look deeper for the underlying causes. And we need to keep this strategy in mind when we look at the SIBO issue. For SIBO to become a problem in your body, you need to have a combination of altered gut motility, low stomach acid, and a poor balance of gut bacteria. The latest studies are crystal clear that these are the real root causes of SIBO. Suffering a lack of motility along with low stomach acid production changes the environment in the gut so that bacteria that normally live down near the colon are able to migrate up toward the stomach. Combine that with multiple rounds of antibiotics, steroids, and drugs over the years, and it creates a perfect recipe for developing SIBO. The following discussion outlines in more detail why these are the three root causes of SIBO-type gut infections.

LOW STOMACH ACID

The first root cause of SIBO relates specifically to what happens in the stomach when we eat. As I pointed out earlier, Americans are taking millions of prescriptions every year to combat heartburn. And although these powerful drugs are very effective at eliminating the symptom of heartburn, they mess up the gut and increase the risk of developing SIBO. Drugs such as Nexium, Prilosec, Prevacid, or other acid-blockers effectively shut off stomach acid production. Additionally, there is mounting research evidence that these drugs have dangerous effects not just on the gut, but on the body as a whole.[15, 16] Far too many Americans are unnecessarily taking these medications, putting their bones, guts, and overall health at risk.

Prescription drugs are not the only cause of stomach acid problems, however. Methylation imbalances, chronic fatigue, fibromyalgia, and many other challenging health conditions that lower energy in the body will drastically affect the digestive system and gut health. Remember that the cells that make stomach acid have a huge number of mitochondria; therefore, anything that poisons our mitochondria impairs the stomach's ability to make hydrochloric acid. Weak mitochondrial function will cause weak digestive function, greatly increasing the risk of developing SIBO. This is especially true in people with methylation problems, who often suffer from impaired mitochondrial function due to a reduced ability to detoxify toxins, hormones, and heavy metals.

At the end of the day, many stomach problems come down to pH levels. When we lack sufficient stomach acid, the food leaving the stomach is far too alkaline. As this less-acidic food enters the small intestine, the pancreas and gallbladder do not release their digestive juices. Without the release of digestive enzymes, bicarbonates, bile, and other juices from the pancreas and gallbladder, the rest of the digestive process is impaired. Not only does this block the absorption of nutrients, but it allows bugs from lower in the bowel to grow and crawl up toward the stomach.

You will remember from chapter 4 that people who take acid-blocking drugs are at an elevated risk of pneumonia and other chronic lung infections. When stomach acid production is weak or nonexistent, the bacteria from the lower small intestine have an easier time moving up toward the stomach and taking hold. Under healthy conditions, the acidity of the stomach as well as the release of bile and pancreatic juices help to prevent SIBO from occurring in the first place.

First, stomach acid kills bacteria that have made their way up near the stomach. And stomach acid is also required to trigger the release of important digestive juices from the pancreas and gallbladder. Second, the digestive enzymes released from the pancreas help to prevent SIBO because they can digest the bacterial cell walls, effectively killing unwanted gut bugs.[17] And, third, the bile released from the gallbladder acts like soap: Just as soap keeps your dishes free of disgusting bacteria and microorganisms, it also helps prevent SIBO in the gut. When bile is released after a meal, it prevents SIBO by washing the bacteria off the walls of the intestine and back down toward the colon.[18] Of course, none of these powerful protective factors help us when our stomach acid has been shut off.

Even something as simple as having low blood sugar can severely impact stomach acid production. As you will learn in chapter 9, skipping meals and allowing the blood sugar to drop quickly lowers stomach acid production significantly. Unfortunately, people with reactive hypoglycemia (the most common type) simply don't digest their food very well. Add to this the fact that, especially as we age, our stomach becomes unable to make adequate amounts of stomach acid, leading to poor digestion. We now know that 30 percent of people over the age of 60 have medically diagnosed hypochlorhydria (they do not produce sufficient hydrochloric acid), highlighting the relationship between age and loss of stomach function.[19] If that weren't enough of a challenge for the aging body, we also lose more of our minerals, leading to a loss of zinc. Zinc is important for stomach function because it is required by the enzyme that makes stomach acid. Many health conditions also involve adrenal stress, where cortisol and aldosterone levels fall. When aldosterone levels drop, the body cannot maintain its supply of sodium and chloride. This leads not only to dizziness and low blood pressure, but it also removes the chloride the body needs to make stomach acid (hydrogen + chloride = hydrochloric acid). Because of these facts, I routinely recommend that everyone over the age of 45 supplement with betaine HCl to assure full assimilation of the nutrients from foods.

ALTERED GUT MOTILITY

The second root cause of SIBO is a dysfunction of the ileocecal valve (ICV), the circular muscle that connects the small and large intestines. In addition to low stomach acid, problems in the ICV help to set the stage for a SIBO infection. As you can see in Figure 6.2, this muscle opens and closes all day long, helping the peristaltic waves of digestion push our food from the kitchen (small intestine) into the bathroom (large intestine). Problems arise when this muscle gets stuck open, and bacteria that normally live only in the colon migrate up toward the stomach, as occurs in SIBO.[20] In support of this idea, research has shown that individuals who have previously had their appendix removed or who have damaged ICVs resulting from surgery are at an elevated risk for SIBO-type gut infections.[21] Surgery can be lifesaving, but it is also like burning a bridge—the tissue will never be the same. When the abdomen and intestines are cut, we develop adhesion, damage nerves and blood vessels, and we often lose function of important structures such as the ICV. Without a healthy ICV, it will be nearly impossible to keep bacteria from crawling from the bathroom into the kitchen. Yuck!

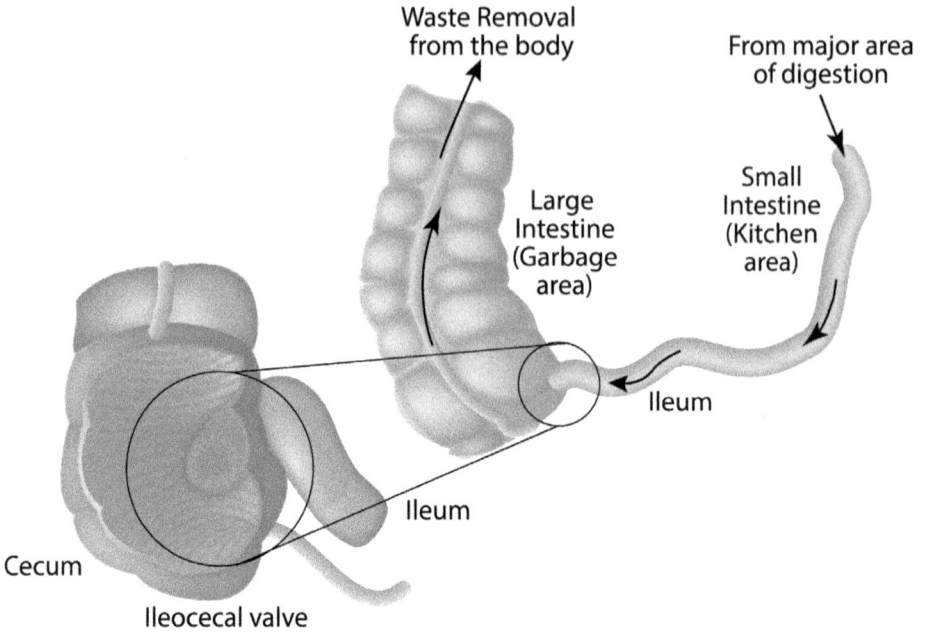

Figure 6.2 - *The ileocecal valve (ICV) connects the small and large intestines, acting as a check-valve to prevent leakage of stool and bacteria from the colon into the small intestine.*

Over the last few years, the connection between the ICV and SIBO has gained a lot of momentum in the research. One major study on this subject was published in 2012 in the *World Journal of Gastroenterology* and perfectly demonstrates this cause-and-effect relationship for developing SIBO. Researchers used a device placed precisely at the junction of the colon and ileum to measure the strength of the muscle contraction in the ICV. Two groups of patients, those with SIBO and those without, were tested during this study. Researchers found that compared to normal subjects without SIBO, those suffering from SIBO had almost no muscle contraction in the ICV.[22] This condition is called an open ileocecal valve, and it allows garbage from the large intestine to leak into the small intestine. The research team summarized its findings by suggesting that many of the symptoms of SIBO—intestinal gas, bloating, and movement of the colonic bacteria into the small intestine—could be related directly to the dysfunction of the ICV. As a chiropractor, I find studies like this to be very exciting.

They prove what many in my profession have known for decades: that treating and adjusting the ICV has a powerful positive effect on the health and function of the digestive system and the body as a whole.

It is important to note that food allergies are another reason why we develop ICV problems. As a culture, we collectively suffer from poor food choices. Just look at the popularity of fast food, processed food, and other junk foods; obviously, we are still in love with food that slowly kills us. Many people's diets consist almost entirely of dairy, gluten, soy, and GMO corn products. You don't have to be a PhD to realize that this type of eating pattern will cause increased levels of inflammation in the ileum and colon, leading to ICV problems. When inflammation develops inside the gut, we often feel pain, bloating, achiness, gas, constipation, or diarrhea. But what also happens, and what many of us don't realize, is that inflammation causes the ICV to stay open. And as the research has shown, when the ICV becomes inflamed and open, it effectively stops working. When we lose ICV function, our risk of developing SIBO goes through the roof!

In addition to ICV problems and food allergy reactions, there is another important cause of altered gut motility: the SIBO problem itself. A balanced, optimum level of bacteria helps keep our bowel muscles working correctly, helping them contract not too fast and not too slow. This bacterial balance keeps us from having diarrhea or constipation, and it keeps the gas and bloating to a bare minimum, making our tummies feel calm and happy. But what happens when the gut is overloaded with way too much bacteria, as we see in SIBO? Excess gut bacteria slows down gut motility, which leads to more gut bacteria. It is a vicious cycle.

Said another way, altered gut motility happens in people with SIBO because it is a major side effect of the infection itself. This raises the question about which comes first: the gut infection that slows down the bowels or slow bowels that create the infection? Although I don't have the answer to that conundrum, I can tell you the research helps us realize that the bacteria itself is likely to blame. In a study in the late 1980s, researchers bred mice with and without gut bacteria. They compared motility and the migrating motor complex of the group of mice with gut bacteria to the germ-free mice (the term "germ-free" denotes the mice that have zero gut bacteria).

These researchers discovered that the germ-free mice had a much faster bowel transit time compared to the mice that had healthy gut bugs.[23] In other words, less gut bacteria translates into faster gut motility. We can see in this study how gut bacteria modulate or influence the function of our digestive tract. We should recognize that having SIBO is the polar opposite of being germ-free—it's a complete overload of gut bacteria. In individuals with a SIBO problem, their bodies have so much bacteria growing where it doesn't belong that it not only creates serious malabsorption and methylation issues, but it also slows down gut motility. As the gut slows down, it becomes harder to push the unwanted bacteria back downhill toward the colon. Thus, the patient with SIBO is trapped, because one of the self-defense mechanisms—gut motility—is slowed when this infection is present. But do not despair, dear reader, because SIBO can be overcome with safe and powerful natural tools found at the end of this chapter.

IMBALANCED GUT FLORA

Having low stomach acid or an irritated and inflamed ICV doesn't automatically mean you have SIBO, but it does mean you are more likely to get it if you don't fix these problems. In addition to these two problems is a third problem that must be discussed as well. The third root cause of SIBO is an imbalance of gut bugs in the intestines. As I said at the beginning of the chapter, there are 10 times as many bugs living in and on us as there are cells in our body. Most of these bugs are healthy and aid in our quest for lasting, radiant health. On the other hand, some aggressive microorganisms threaten our health and increase the likelihood that we will develop gut infections like SIBO.

Inside of everyone's gut are some bad bugs; they are always present, even in a healthy gut ecosystem. They include viruses, yeasts and fungi like *Candida albicans*, and even parasites and worms! (Worms are actually very common; according to the CDC, about 26 percent of all adults worldwide have a roundworm infection in their gut.[24]) And it's this way for a reason: the bad bugs help the immune system stay vigilant and strong. When we talk about imbalanced gut flora as a cause of SIBO, we really mean the problems that arise when our good bugs disappear and the gangster bugs take over.

THE DIET PROBLEM

Let's look at the modern American diet and then move on to examine how antibiotics destroy our delicate gut environment. High sugar, high fat diets are proven to increase your risk of cancer, heart disease, depression, and a long list of other diseases. Although almost everyone knows that eating junk food diets ultimately leads to diabetes and clogged arteries, few people are aware that these diets drastically change the gut microbes as well.

NOTE: So much research is coming out showing how gut bacteria changes our health that I don't have room to cover it all here. I would recommend that readers who are interested in further study on this topic to get a copy of the excellent book Brain Maker by Dr. David Perlmutter. He does an excellent job summarizing much of the current research in this area.

Just like different animals in the forest have different dietary requirements, so, too, do our gut bugs. In general, the health-sustaining gut bacteria such as *Lactobacillus* and *Bifidobacteria* survive on fiber and nutrients from vegetables. These bugs are especially adapted to eating the parts of plants that we cannot digest. They eat our waste and excrete nutrients, vitamins, and amino acids that enrich our bodies. It's a beautiful symbiotic relationship. But when we eat the "standard American diet," the balance in our gut is threatened. And as the balance of our gut bugs change, so, too, does our risk of developing SIBO.

Modern, processed, junk-food diets are feeding the gangster bugs while starving out the happy, hard-working ones. As one example of this problem, consider a 2013 study published in the journal *Nature Immunology*. Researchers demonstrated that pathogenic, disease-causing strains of *E. coli* prefer to eat carbohydrates that other healthy bacteria do not eat or use for fuel.[25] In other words, the more refined carbohydrates we put into our gut, the more we feed the gangster SIBO-causing bugs. As we feed the bad bugs, we are starving the healthy bacteria of the fiber and other ingredients they need to survive. As the years go by, this high sugar, high fat diet and lifestyle will promote the dominance of aggressive gut bacteria and increase the odds of developing SIBO.

Modern junk-food diets provide the perfect fuel for a SIBO infection and other intestinal bugs like *Candida albicans* to grow rapidly. *Candida* is a type of yeast organism that must use fermentation to survive. And no discussion of SIBO would be complete without mentioning chronic yeast issues. Whether resulting from antibiotics, stress, or poor dietary choices, aggressive yeast species create fermentation in the gut, often causing bloating, gas, pain, and malabsorption. Yeast also produces aldehydes and alcohols that impair brain focus and concentration, and lead to serious problems in the methylation cycle (more on this in chapter 7). Many common foods including fruit, refined sugar, processed carbohydrates, and fermented foods provide an excellent fuel for yeast to grow. Although some yeast in our gut is completely healthy, many people are walking around with way too much *Candida* and other fungi living in their digestive tracts. These hidden yeast infections don't cause SIBO per se, but they contribute to the hostile environment, the inflammation, and the malabsorption that accompanies SIBO.

Gut bacteria, like yeast, also use the process of fermentation to produce energy and survive. When we have a SIBO infection, the more fermentable foods we eat, the worse the infection becomes. Since SIBO is an overgrowth of bacteria, logic would suggest that starving this mass of bacteria would be helpful in treating it. And this is precisely the reasoning behind using a FODMAP (which stands for fermentable oligosaccharides, disaccharides, monosaccharides, and polyols) diet to help treat SIBO: it helps to cull the excess bacteria. Because of the close relationship between yeast and bacteria, I find that patients must often treat both at the same time. (You can find much more on the FODMAP diet and how to use it in the back of this book. As you will see in the protocol section, the genius solution for ridding the body of SIBO is very similar to the solution for getting rid of *Candida*.) Although the modern diet is certainly at fault for creating an overgrowth of bad bugs, the overuse of antibiotics in our society takes this problem to a whole new level.

THE ANTIBIOTIC PROBLEM

Although food and diet choices are major contributors to the SIBO problem, many cases of SIBO are caused by antibiotics. These dangerous drugs don't just kill "bad" bacteria; they also kill the "good" bacteria and make it more likely that the surviving bugs grow aggressively and take over the intestines. Without the healthy bugs in our gut, we don't benefit from all the nutrients in our food, our immune system becomes progressively inflamed, and we can suffer for years with chronic leaky gut problems. By taking antibiotics, we may make the symptom go away temporarily, but we create even bigger issues later on.

Although the promise of rapid, side effect-free treatment gets the attention of both doctors and patients, using antibiotics to treat SIBO isn't well supported in the research—at least from a long-term perspective. True, many studies show that antibiotics such as Rifaximin and others greatly reduce the symptoms of SIBO and IBS over a few days and weeks.[26, 27, 28, 29] Despite the evidence that antibiotics can be used to treat SIBO, a closer review of the data shows that using them isn't actually a wise choice. The current research shows that after treating SIBO with antibiotic therapy, more than half of all cases of SIBO return in nine months' time.[30] Not only that, but many of the studies that show antibiotics are helpful for SIBO consistently report that only 50 percent of patients will see any relief, temporary or otherwise, by using high-dose antibiotic therapy. So this leaves you with a 50 percent chance of getting short-term relief but a 100 percent chance of hurting your gut in the long term. The problem is this: Antibiotics never improve gut function, only gut symptoms, and a poorly functioning gut is the main reason why SIBO occurs in the first place! Remember that antibiotics don't alter the gut environment in a positive way and do nothing to heal and prevent SIBO effectively in the long term.

Just as a forest fire destroys the trees on the side of a mountain, antibiotics kill bacteria. But not all bacteria are killed when antibiotics are given. Mostly, the good guys—*Lactobacillis* and *Bifidobacteria*—are killed, but the aggressive, antibiotic-resistant strains usually survive. On a fire-scorched mountainside, weeds and invasive plants grow with abandon, since they no longer face competition for sunlight, nutrition, and space. It is exactly the same in the gut. We now know that even a single round of antibiotics is strong enough to alter our digestive tract for months.

To highlight this point, I'll again turn to the peer-reviewed literature. A fascinating study published in 2015 demonstrates that even the smallest doses of antibiotics will cause long-term damage to the gut microbiome. Researchers point out how antibiotics are used routinely as a prophylaxis—a tool to prevent an infection rather than to treat an infection—and rightly suggest that this is leading to dangerous antibiotic-resistant bacteria. And although no one wants to go through surgery and get a life-threatening infection, data shows that using antibiotics as a preventative measure is starting to backfire. Researchers found that even a single round of antibiotics upsets the diversity of the digestive tract, killing off healthy bacteria for several months while increasing the likelihood of developing antibiotic resistance in the future.[31] All that damage occurs after a single round that typically lasts three to seven days. I routinely meet patients who have had more than 50 doses of antibiotics over their lifetime—we have no idea how much damage that causes to our bodies.

With so many prescriptions for antibiotics being filled in our society, it is no wonder that SIBO is becoming more common. Studies show that when antibiotics kill the good bacteria, the aggressive bugs gain access to more nutrition and grow faster. When aggressive gut "weeds" begin to grow, they don't always stay in one place; they often start to spread into the upper small intestine. This is how antibiotics give rise to SIBO over time. Of course, when we are healthy, the aggressive bacteria are kept in check by our good flora. Research shows that when certain *Lactobacillus* species are present in the gut, they prevent pain, gas, and bloating associated with IBS and SIBO.[32] The good bacteria make it harder for the bad bacteria to survive, and we reap the benefits of this biological warfare. It is no wonder that millions of people are suffering with IBS and SIBO-like problems, given the overconsumption of powerful antibiotic medications. If antibiotics are used "just in case" during every medical intervention, someday there will be no antibiotics left that can actually save lives.

Bacteria learn how to avoid being killed by antibiotics through the process of epigenetics. You'll remember that epigenetics is the process our cells use to change our genetic expression based on the environment inside our bodies. And while your genius body uses this fascinating and empowering science of epigenetics to improve health, it can also work to destroy health. The environment is a two-way street. If we work to produce healthy environments, then we get healthy genetic responses, not just in our own cells but in the cells of the microbes upon which we depend for life. Conversely, if we toxify our bodies and pollute our bowels with exposure to antibiotics, GMO foods, and other toxic inputs, we can expect a negative genetic response. Without treating the root cause and improving the environment inside the gut, we cannot expect our body to rid itself fully of chronic infections like SIBO. If we have a SIBO-style gut infection, everything we eat will be a potential trigger of our immune system and our adrenal fight-or-flight reflex. When SIBO is present, we unknowingly create a perfect storm for messed up methylation all over our bodies.

CONCLUSION

The research discussed in this chapter highlights the fact that SIBO gut infections create methylation problems. Having too much folic acid can create a methylation imbalance, and unmetabolized folic acid is a known side effect of a SIBO problem. Many patients with digestive symptoms such as bloating, reflux, gas, and abdominal pain of a chronic nature are suffering from some form of SIBO. Even if we avoid fortified foods and high doses of folic acid, just having SIBO means we can still be absorbing folic acid directly from the gut itself, creating a methylation issue throughout the body.

SIBO is a growing problem that is caused by chronic stress, bad food choices, and side effects of commonly used medications. The standard of care in the United States still relies heavily on antibiotics and PPIs to treat gastrointestinal complaints. If all you are trying to do is make the symptoms go away, these approaches work well. Ask anyone who takes Nexium or omeprazole for heartburn, and they will tell you how well it "makes the burning go away." And we can't argue that point: if you shut off acid production completely in the stomach, there will be no burning.

Unfortunately, these toxic substances also make it very difficult to absorb nutrients from your food while they simultaneously promote the growth of pathogenic bacteria.

Research now shows that dangerous and unnecessary drugs used to treat gastrointestinal complaints are responsible for causing SIBO. The fact of the matter is that we overuse drugs in our society. Whenever drugs are used, in almost every case, there exists a natural alternative that works often better than the drug, that has zero to few side effects, and that promotes rather than hinders our overall health.

I have been helping many patients heal their guts naturally and balance their genetics. After helping patients with many difficult and challenging problems, I have learned to treat the gut first, making sure to clear out the gut infections before embarking on supporting methylation. Through rigorous trial and error, I have learned that until the gut is working properly, there cannot be methylation balance. By learning about the methylation science and following the advice in this book, you can also get great results! And as you will see again and again throughout the remainder of this book, gut health really makes the biggest difference to our genes, our health, and our lives.

SIBO PROTOCOL

The protocol for treating SIBO is simple, but difficult to follow. Treating SIBO effectively requires two basic things: starving the bacteria by not eating fermentable food and killing the bacteria with natural herbs and compounds. This is what makes the protocol hard to follow, because a lot of our favorite foods are easily fermentable by bacteria. If we eat fermentable foods while trying to cure SIBO, our healing process will take much, much longer. The best SIBO diet we have found was compiled by Dr. Allison Siebecker and can be downloaded from her website free of charge. You will find information about her website and the Siebecker FODMAP/SCD diet in appendix D.

Another issue with SIBO treatment is to avoid probiotics, especially in the first 3 to 4 weeks. A mountain of evidence shows how helpful probiotics are to our bodies, but remember that too much of a good thing can be a bad thing. Many SIBO patients we work with report bloating/discomfort while taking probiotics, and for that reason we don't put them in this protocol. If you choose to use probiotics after the first month, start slow with a low dose product such as UltraBiotic Daily from Nutridyn at 1 capsule per day.

RECOMMENDED LAB TESTING:

I recommend the Routine Blood Tests and the Organic Acid Test (OAT) in appendix B for assessing the full extent of the SIBO and related issues. Often the OAT will clearly show SIBO problems, but in some cases the OAT will miss it. In cases where SIBO is suspected from symptoms, but the OAT is clear, it is appropriate to then test for SIBO directly with the SIBO Breath Test listed in appendix B. To make full use of the information in this book, I recommend following the instructions found in appendix A to get your own detailed genetic report.

SIBO PROTOCOL:

To remove the unwanted bacteria/parasites/yeast thoroughly from the intestines, it is helpful to use a variety of bug-killing supplements. By rotating the products, there is less chance that the bacteria will become resistant to the treatment. The goal is to rotate between Groups One, Two, and Three every 4 days. For example, for the first 4 days take the Group One bug killers, then on day 5 stop taking Group One and switch to taking Group Two, and finally on day 9 switch from Group Two to Group Three. Rotate back to Group One products on day 13 and so on.

This rotation has proven helpful for many of our patients with chronic SIBO issues. Most people see results by 4 weeks, but stubborn cases of SIBO may require an extended period of treatment from 3 to 6 months. Remember, we are all individuals.

Group One

Spectrum AR – 1 softgel 3 times per day with meals. These aromatic oils work as well as gold standard antibiotics at killing bad bugs, yet avoid the negative side effects of antibiotic treatment. Cleanses the bowel of bacteria/viruses/yeast/parasites.† (Nutridyn)

Spectrum BR – 2 tablets 3 times per day with meals. Oils of berberine are very effective for removing more bacteria/viruses/yeast/parasites from the GI tract.† (Nutridyn)

Group Two

Urinary Cleanse – 1 full dropper 3 times per day with meals. High levels of Uva Ursi which is an excellent herb for killing bacteria/yeast/fungi. Uva Ursi also has a preferential effect on the urinary tract and is useful for killing pathogens irritating the bladder and kidney.† (Nutridyn)

GSE Pro – 1 capsule 3 times per day with meals. Grapefruit seed extract (GSE) is a highly concentrated fungal and microbial balancing extract. Grapefruit seed extract exerts these effects within the gastrointestinal tract, promoting healthy microflora and gut ecology.† (Nutridyn)

Group Three

Micro Eze – 1 capsule 3 times per day with meals. Ayervedic ingredients to help kill gut infections and promote the growth of healthy intestinal flora through three potent ingredients. Neem extract, vidanga extract, and *Mimosa pudica* extract work to promote detoxification and support a healthy gut microbiome.† (Nutridyn)

B-Cleanse – 3 capsules 2 times per day with meals. Blend of six different antimicrobials to help cleanse the GI tract of unwanted and excessive bacteria/viruses/yeast/parasites and provide a broad spectrum therapeutic effect.† (Nutridyn)

In addition, patients are advised to use the following supplements to help improve the function of their upper GI tract and reduce leaky gut symptoms while taking bug-killing supplements.

SIBO UPPER GI SUPPORT PROTOCOL:

HCl Support – HCl stomach acid that supports digestion and helps break down food. Take this product at the end of the meal. To find out what dose is best for you, see the HCl stomach acid instructions page.† (Nutridyn)

Pan 5X – Pancreatic enzymes will help you break down your food. Take 1 or 2 capsules 5 minutes before meals/shakes/snacks. Will improve digestion and absorption of nutrients.† (Nutridyn)

Stress Essentials Relax – 2 capsules 3 times per day with meals. Helps to support glutathione production in the liver and provides high doses of taurine to improve bile flow; also provides B6, which is necessary for oxalate detoxification inside the liver.| (Nutridyn)

D3 10,000 with K2 – 1 softgel per day with a meal. Provides numerous benefits to the health and function of the GI tract, and SIBO patients are chronically low in fat-soluble vitamins like D3.† (Nutridyn)

L-Glutamine Powder – 2 tablespoons 3 times per day with or without meals. Glutamine is the main fuel source for the cells which line our intestines. This product provides concentrated levels of L-glutamine to help reduce leaky gut symptoms.†‡ (Nutridyn)

---

†This statement has not been evaluated by the FDA. This product is not intended to diagnose, treat, cure, or prevent any disease. The information provided in this book is intended for your general knowledge only and is not a substitute for professional medical advice or treatment for specific medical conditions. You should not use this information to diagnose or treat a health problem or disease without consulting with a qualified healthcare provider. Please consult your healthcare provider with any questions or concerns you may have regarding your condition. Never disregard professional medical advice or delay in seeking it because of something you have read in this book.

COFFEE ENEMA SUPPORT:

And, finally, for a more effective SIBO treatment protocol, I recommend using coffee enemas to speed clearance of dead bacteria from your colon and to help detoxify the liver in the process. You can find instructions for how to perform coffee enemas in appendix D. For patients who are going through SIBO or other gut-infection protocols, I typically recommend one coffee enema per day for a week, then three times per week for one month. Coffee enemas are safe and well tolerated, and they can be safely used for extended periods of time.

Organo Gold® Gourmet Black Ganoderma Coffee – This is the recommended coffee for coffee enemas. The advantage of instant coffee is that you don't have to wait for the boiling water to cool down before performing the enema. I have wasted hours trying to get the boiled coffee to the correct body temperature before I realized that instant coffee from Organo Gold® solves that problem. You can find ordering information for this enema coffee in appendix C.

HIATAL HERNIA AND ICV SUPPORT:

I believe that every SIBO patient has low stomach acid, poor pancreatic function, poor gallbladder function, a hiatal hernia, and an ileocecal valve (ICV) issue, until proven otherwise. Patients are advised to find an Applied Kinesiology–certified doctor who can help restore function to their ICV and fix their hiatal hernia. You can find such a doctor near you by going to the ICAKUSA website recommended in appendix E.

REFERENCES

1. Bianconi, E., A. Piovesan, F. Facchin, et al. An estimation of the number of cells in the human body. *Ann Hum Biol.* (2013) 40(6): 463-71. Epub 2013 Jul 5.

2. NIH Human Microbiome Project defines normal bacterial makeup of the body. National Institutes of Health website. www.nih.gov/news/health/jun2012/nhgri-13.htm. Published on June 13, 2012. Accessed January 25, 2016.

3. Hoffbrand, A.V., D.G. Weir. The history of folic acid. *Br J Haematol.* (2001) 113(3): 579-89.

4. Rong, N., J. Selhub, B.R. Goldin, et al. Bacterially synthesized folate in rat large intestine is incorporated into host tissue folyl polyglutamates. *J Nutr.* (1991) 121(12): 1955-59. PMID: 1941259

5. D'Aimmo, M.R., P. Mattarelli, B. Biavati, et al. The potential of bifidobacteria as a source of natural folate. *J Appl Microbiol.* (2012) 112(5): 975-84.

6. Strozzi, G.P., L. Mogna. Quantification of folic acid in human feces after administration of *Bifidobacterium* probiotic strains. *J Clin Gastroenterol.* (2008) 42 Suppl 3 Pt 2: S179-84.

7. Bermingham, A., J.P. Derrick. The folic acid biosynthesis pathway in bacteria: evaluation of potential for antibacterial drug discovery. *Bioessays.* (2002) 24(7): 637-48.

8. Dukowicz, A.C., B.E. Lacy, G.M. Levine. Small intestinal bacterial overgrowth: a comprehensive review. *Gastroenterol Hepatol (N Y).* (2007) 3(2): 112-22.

9. Christensen, K.E., L.G. Mikael, K.Y. Leung, et al. High folic acid consumption leads to pseudo-MTHFR deficiency, altered lipid metabolism, and liver injury in mice. *Am J Clin Nutr.* (2015) 101(3): 646-58.

10. Henderson, G.B. Folate-binding proteins. *Annu Rev Nutr.* (1990) 10: 319-35.

11. Pyleris, F., E.J. Giamarellos-Bourboulis, D. Izivras, et al. The prevalence of overgrowth by aerobic bacteria in the small intestine by small bowel culture: relationship with irritable bowel syndrome. *Dig Dis Sci.* (2012) 57(5): 1321-29.

12. Pimentel, M., R.P. Gunsalus, S.C. Rao, et al. Methanogens in Human Health and Disease. *Am J Gastroenterol Suppl* (2012) 1: 28-33.

13. Tong, M., I. McHardy, P. Ruegger, et al. Reprogramming of gut microbiome energy metabolism by the FUT2 Crohn's disease risk polymorphism. *ISME J.* (2014) 8(11): 2193-2206.

14. Lewis, Z.T., S.M. Totten, J.T. Smilowitz, et al. Maternal fucosyltransferase 2 status affects the gut bifidobacterial communities of breastfed infants. *Microbiome.* (2015) 3: 13.

15. Lombardo, L., M. Foti, O. Ruggia, et al. Increased incidence of small intestinal bacterial overgrowth during proton pump inhibitor therapy. *Clin Gastroenterol Hepatol.* (2010) 8(6): 504-8.

16. Compare, D., L. Pica, A. Rocco, et al. Effects of long-term PPI treatment on producing bowel symptoms and SIBO. *Eur J Clin Invest*. (2011) 41(4): 380-86.

17. Bures, J., J. Cyrany, D. Kohoutova, et al. Small intestinal bacterial overgrowth syndrome. *World J Gastroenterol*. (2010) 16(24): 2978-90.

18. Monte, M.J., J.J. Marin, A. Antelo, et al. Bile acids: chemistry, physiology, and pathophysiology. *World J Gastroenterol*. (2009) 15(7): 804-16.

19. Schinke, T., A.F. Schilling, A. Baranowsky, et al. Impaired gastric acidification negatively affects calcium homeostasis and bone mass. *Nat Med*. (2009) 15(6): 674-81.

20. Roland, B.C., M.M. Ciarleglio, J.O. Clarke, et al. Low ileocecal valve pressure is significantly associated with small intestinal bacterial overgrowth (SIBO). *Dig Dis Sci*. (2014) 59(6): 1269-77.

21. Schatz, R.A., Q. Zhang, N. Lodhia, et al. Predisposing factors for positive D-Xylose breath test for evaluation of small intestinal bacterial overgrowth: a retrospective study of 932 patients. *World J Gastroenterol*. (2015) 21(15): 4574-82.

22. Miller, L.S., A.K. Vegesna, A.M. Sampath, et al. Ileocecal valve dysfunction in small intestinal bacterial overgrowth: A pilot study. *World J Gastroenterol*. (2012) 18(46): 6801-8.

23. Caenepeel, P., J. Janssens, G. Vantrappen, et al. Interdigestive myoelectric complex in germ-free rats. *Dig Dis Sci*. (1989) 34(8): 1180-84.

24. Parasites – Ascariasis. Center for Disease Control website. www.cdc.gov/parasites/ascariasis/index.html. Published on January 10, 2013. Accessed February 6, 2016.

25. Kamada, N., G.Y. Chen, N. Inohara, et al. Control of pathogens and pathobionts by the gut microbiota. *Nat Immunol*. (2013) 14(7): 685-90.

26. Pimentel, M., E.J. Chow, and H.C. Lin. Eradication of small intestinal bacterial overgrowth reduces symptoms of irritable bowel syndrome. *Am J Gastroenterol*. (2000) 95(12): 3503-6.

27. Majewski, M., S.C. Reddymasu, S. Sostarich, et al. Efficacy of rifaximin, a nonabsorbed oral antibiotic, in the treatment of small intestinal bacterial overgrowth. *Am J Med Sci*. (2007) 333(5): 266-70.

28. Furnari, M., A. Parodi, L. Gemignani, et al. Clinical trial: the combination of rifaximin with partially hydrolysed guar gum is more effective than rifaximin alone in eradicating small intestinal bacterial overgrowth. *Aliment Pharmacol Ther*. (2010) 32(8): 1000-6.

29. Lauritano, E.C., M. Gabrielli, E. Scarpellini, et al. Antibiotic therapy in small intestinal bacterial overgrowth: rifaximin versus metronidazole. *Eur Rev Med Pharmacol Sci*. (2009) 13(2): 111-16.

30. Lauritano, E.C., M. Gabrielli, E. Scarpellini, et al. Small intestinal bacterial overgrowth recurrence after antibiotic therapy. *Am J Gastroenterol*. (2008) 103(8): 2031-35.

31. Zaura, E., B.W. Brandt, M.J. Teixeira de Mattos, et al. Same Exposure but Two Radically Different

Responses to Antibiotics: Resilience of the Salivary Microbiome versus Long-Term Microbial Shifts in Feces. *MBio*. (2015) 6(6): e01693-1715.

32. Bixquert Jiménez, M. Treatment of irritable bowel syndrome with probiotics. An etiopathogenic approach at last? *Rev Esp Enferm Dig*. (2009) 101(8): 553-64.

7.

GUT ORIGINS OF METHYLATION PROBLEMS

In all chaos there is a cosmos, in all disorder a secret order.

—Carl Jung

So far in our quest, we have seen how low stomach acid, high oxalates, and small intestine bacterial overgrowth can interfere with the methylation cycle and put our health in jeopardy. But we aren't even halfway through this journey of connecting the dots between our gut, our genes, our brain, and our health. To understand truly how our genius body works, you have to delve even further into how the chemistry of the gut impacts the chemistry of every cell in your body. You are about to see how compounds produced by bacteria and yeast within your digestive system can slow detoxification and make a mess of your methylation cycle. You are about to learn the amazing truth of how the bugs in your gut interfere with and influence the genetic pathways inside your body.

Let's begin this effort with a very important question: Have you ever considered that your gut microorganisms can influence your genes? Although that question might sound strange at first, it is exactly what the latest research is showing. Consider, for example, that according to Dr. Steven Gundry, there are 10 times as many foreign cells in our gut than we have cells in our body. Dr. Gundry also points out that due to the large number of bacteria, viruses, fungi, and parasites, our GI tract contains 100 times the amount of genetic material (DNA and RNA) than we carry in the rest our body—that's two orders of magnitude![1] What he is sharing with us is that if you want to optimize your genes, you must optimize your gut. And if you follow the advice in this book, you can do just that!

If the gut carries so much genetic material, it will have a major impact on the function of our own methylation-related pathways. It is apparent that the microorganisms in our gut determine more than just how well we digest food; the compounds released by the microorganisms in the gut are known to influence our brain chemistry, hormones, blood sugar, sleep cycle, and much more. Far from being quiet neighbors living in our intestines, gut microbes have a huge impact on the function and expression of our genes.

This chapter highlights three nasty gut toxins that can cause damage to your methylation cycle and disrupt your detoxification pathways. In the chapters to follow, I will explain how our genetic SNPs in the COMT, MAO, MTHFR, and related pathways lead to increased levels of adrenaline and dopamine, which in turn lead to increases in pain and anxiety. Anxiety is something we have all felt, but many people are trapped in a world where they cannot find peace because of constant worry, panic, and pain. I routinely work with patients from all over the world who are stuck in a stress-mess, anxiety fest state of mind. And the common denominator in all these cases is a genetic imbalance that affects how their bodies detoxify stress chemicals—dopamine, epinephrine, and norepinephrine.

SNPs of Concern

As you learned in the SIBO chapter, many methylation genes are very sensitive to gut problems. These genes take it on the chin when the gut has gone awry:

- *COMT* – Catechol-O-methyltransferase
- *MAO* – Monoamine oxidase
- *MTR* – Methionine synthase
- *SULT* – Phenol sulfotransferase
- *ALDH* – Aldehyde dehydrogenase
- *ADH* – Alcohol dehydrogenase
- *ALR* – Aldehyde reductase

Although those genetic variations we carry certainly do influence our perception of pain and our feelings of anxiety, another part of the story needs to be mentioned first: the gut origin of anxiety and methylation problems. It might not make sense at first glance that gut bacteria can influence your methylation cycle and change your mood, but that is what the research now shows. And as you will learn in chapter 8, yeasts and gut bacteria have their own methylation cycles. In other words, those nutrients that help optimize your methylation cycle so you can grow and repair also help gut microbes grow and repair. This is a nutritional double-edged sword!

GUT BUGS AND VITAMIN MONSTERS

I consistently meet patients who, in their search for answers, have discovered the powerful process of methylation. Many of these individuals take methylation support vitamins such as folate, B12, and more, to try to support their health and increase their well-being. Much to their surprise, they experience a severe flare-up and worsening of their symptoms when they take methylated B vitamins. This makes them scared, anxious, and confused about how to get better. And my heart goes out to them, because I know that it is frustrating that something that should help you feel better actually makes you feel worse. I have to remind my patients that the body doesn't make mistakes. Our biology is pure genius, so if we see a side effect from something that should work, we need to search to determine why the body doesn't accept it, yet. And, of course, as you probably guessed, the gut is the place to start that search.

When you take methylation vitamins, it is like you're dumping fertilizer into your gut. You expect that the fertilizer, the B vitamins, will be distributed throughout your body. Unfortunately, however, that is not the case, because the gut bacteria and microorganisms get a chance to eat them first. When patients tell me they aren't getting better despite a perfect diet and healthy supplements, I know that the problem is in their gut!

Not only do gut bacteria produce vitamins that you need, they also produce toxins that disturb your methylation cycle and lead to anxiety, tension, insomnia, pain, fatigue, and brain fog. Taking methylation support vitamins can save your life, and I have a long list of patients who have benefited enormously from the right blend of methyl nutrients. However, if your gut is dumping toxins into your body when you take vitamins, then it will slow your progress considerably.

Healthy gut bacteria aid in absorbing vitamins, while unhealthy gut bugs get in the way. It's just that simple. By now, you should be able to see how your gut, brain, and the methylation cycle are all connected in a beautiful, genius fashion.

When aggressive bacteria and yeasts eat your "fertilizer" first, they grow stronger, while you become progressively malnourished. This is a main reason why people who take vitamins and eat healthy foods may have symptom flare-ups or may not be getting better. It means something in the gut is eating all that fertilizer and making them sick. It could be a parasite they picked up on a trip to Mexico or a nasty type of bacteria that landed in their gut after a bout of food poisoning. Or it could be a gut imbalance they developed after living through a prolonged stressful event, such as a divorce, starting a new business, or starting a family. A perfect example of this problem can be found by reviewing how SIBO impacts the methylation cycle:

- SIBO causes iron-deficient anemia, low protein, and malnutrition in general.

- SIBO makes it hard to gain weight and slows growth in children.

- SIBO increases blood folic acid and folate levels, interfering with MTHFR pathways.

- SIBO decreases absorption of B12 and fatty vitamins such as A, D, E, and K, leading to poor methylation and chronic disease.

Now, obviously, SIBO is a severe form of this problem, but it does illustrate the point. When our gut is imbalanced and overgrown with bacteria and yeast, we simply cannot optimize our health or our genes. I don't want you to get the idea that gut microbes and bacteria can only harm us. The truth is, without the proper bacteria and microorganisms in our gut, we cannot survive. We absolutely depend on those organisms to provide our bodies with nutrients to create health. So although microbes and bacteria are necessary for health, anything that is good can become toxic if it begins to get out of balance. And this gut imbalance is the driving force behind so many symptoms that make people with methylation issues chronically sick.

THE BIG THREE MICROBIAL BYPRODUCTS THAT IMPAIR METHYLATION

Three very important methylation-destroying gut toxins can increase anxiety, pain, insomnia, brain fog, headaches, and more: phenols, aromatic amino acids, and aldehydes. These chemicals, which are pooped out by the bacteria and yeasts in our intestines, easily find their way into our liver and the rest of our body. And when we consider how these bacterial compounds produced in the gut influence our methylation cycle, we can see that gut infections can halt progress in someone who is trying to fix methylation problems. You are about to discover all the different ways phenols, aromatic amino acids, and aldehydes can impact your methylation cycle and wreck your health.

PHENOL COMPOUNDS

To understand how bacteria mess with our methylation cycle, we need to learn about phenol. Phenols are volatile chemical compounds that come from plants and bacteria. Everyone has phenols in their body; they are a normal part of our gut environment.

Phenols in the gut are also called volatile organic compounds, or VOCs. You've likely seen this phrase when shopping for paint or reading about toxins released from petroleum products such as vinyl flooring. It is fascinating to realize that the same chemicals that pollute our external environment are also found in our internal environment. It's not a question of whether we are exposed to phenols; it is a question of how many toxic phenols we have to deal with. Everyone has a different tolerance to volatile organic compounds, aka organic acids, before symptoms develop. Some phenols, such as resveratrol and green tea catechins, have enormous health benefits. I use these compounds regularly with patients with excellent results. But just because some phenols give us benefits doesn't mean that all phenols are helpful. In fact, phenols in high amounts can be a big problem for the brain, liver, and methylation cycle in general.

Because they have similar chemical shapes, the phenolic compounds such as those produced by our gut bacteria compete with estrogen, adrenaline, and dopamine for metabolism through the COMT phase II detoxification pathway. By slowing down the COMT pathway, phenols increase the half-life of estrogen and catecholamines, the stress neurotransmitters known as dopamine, norepinephrine, and epinephrine. Therefore, if the imbalanced gut is causing too many phenols to leak into our body, it will slow the clearance of estrogen and stress hormones. I recognize not everyone reading this studies genetics and biochemistry, so all these pathways and chemicals can get a little confusing. So to make these points a little clearer, I'll explain further.

Estrogens, reproductive hormones, are removed from our body mainly by the gallbladder. Any problem that increases estrogens, such as a gut-phenol issue, will put a lot of stress on the gallbladder as it tries to manage the excess estrogen. We know that high estrogen is a trigger for gallbladder issues to start, which is why women experience the vast majority of gallbladder problems. That is a problem that will develop even without inherited polymorphisms in the COMT, MTHFR, and related pathways. In other words, you don't have to have problem genes to experience gallbladder issues; all you really need is a gut problem loading up your liver with phenols. That will create the same situation as having a genetic imbalance. And if you happen to have a genetic imbalance as well as a gut phenol problem, your body will truly struggle to create optimum health. The phenols compete with estrogen for detoxification, which causes estrogen levels to build up. In this way, the hormonal system in the body is greatly influenced by the bacteria in the gut. (You will learn more about fascinating connections between hormones and methylation in chapter 12.) I wish phenol problems were limited to messing with hormones, but that would miss another important aspect to this story.

As you are beginning to realize, bacteria aren't just silent neighbors living in our gut. They can impact not only our hormone levels, as I have just described, but they also change how we tolerate the stress of daily life. These bacterial waste products have the capacity to influence our methylation cycle greatly by inhibiting the breakdown of catecholamines. These bacteria-derived phenol compounds increase the half-life of adrenaline and catecholamines in our bodies. The longer the half-life of a chemical, the longer it will be active. Because gut-based phenols slow the detoxification of catecholamines, they significantly reduce how much stress we can handle. The problem here is that interfering with the detoxification of adrenaline will cause it to build up inside the body. And you don't need to be a doctor to realize that excess adrenaline is a bad idea. Individuals with this gut-based issue often experience symptoms such as insomnia, anxiety, worry, and chronic pain. I am sure many of you reading this consider these symptoms to be very familiar. Despite changing their diet and taking supplements, many people with phenol issues cannot find relief from symptoms like these without treating the gut-based problem first.

The key point to understand is that phenols are a normal part of the gut environment. Even healthy bacteria produce these chemicals on a daily basis. Recent research has shown that many common species of gut bacteria such as *Bifidobacterium, Clostridium difficile* (*C. diff*), *Escherichia coli* (*E. coli*), and *Lactobacillus* produce phenols, leading our bodies to excrete from 50 to 100mg of volatile phenols each day.[2] Understand that phenols are a normal part of our gut environment and they always leak into our body to some degree; this is a natural and healthy process and no cause for alarm. Yet when the bacteria get out of hand, the amount of phenols the body must detoxify increases dramatically. Since each phenol molecule from the gut will have to be processed through our methylation and sulfation detoxification pathways, excess gut phenols will have a serious impact on our body's biochemistry. And the last thing we all need is slowed detoxification and methylation.

To illustrate this concept, we turn to research that is more than 40 years old. In the first study published in 1970, researchers injected benzoic acid (a type of phenol) into mice and measured how much it slowed down the activity of COMT. Incredibly, after injecting phenols into the mice, their liver COMT function slowed by 100 percent for more than 45 minutes.[3] In the second study published in 1973, researchers confirmed these findings when they determined that a phenol called pyrogallol also effectively inhibited COMT function inside the body.[4] What this scientific research proves is that phenols are capable of interfering with our methylation cycle and detoxification pathways. This is exactly how imbalances in the gut can change genetic responses inside of our body.

As anyone who understands drug metabolism will tell you, if you increase the half-life of a chemical you are going to increase the length of time it will be effective. In other words, if you block the breakdown of adrenaline, dopamine, and estrogen by slowing the COMT pathways, you will create a stronger stress reaction. This will make an individual less tolerant of stress, since each time the body releases adrenaline, it is staying active far longer than normal. All the intolerance to life's various stressors can be traced back to how the gut bacteria is influencing our genetics.

Because most of you reading this book aren't scientists or doctors, I think a metaphor can help clarify this idea. If the gut is producing a lot of phenols (during SIBO or other gut infections), the body cannot detox stress hormones and estrogens very well, because the phenols sit in the same parking space in the COMT enzyme as adrenaline, dopamine, and estrogen. High phenol levels from the gut can lead to pain, anxiety, insomnia, fatigue, low thyroid, fibroids, endometriosis, obesity, and more, just by interfering with the COMT pathway and putting excess pressure on other sulfur-based phase II detoxification systems. But that is not all that gut-derived phenols can do.

Phenols are also metabolized through the sulfation pathway, and processing phenols can lower sulfate levels.[5] The SULT1A1 and SULT1A2 genes are responsible for taking a toxin, neurotransmitter, bile acid, or hormone, and gluing it to a molecule of sulfate.[6] This sulfate transfer is important to phase II detox. All phenols, whether they come from the gut or the diet, must be processed through the SULT pathway in the liver. When phenols are metabolized this way, they will permanently remove sulfate from the body; the more phenols get into the body, the more sulfate is needed to remove them. And as you learned in chapter 5, sulfate is often lacking in people with imbalanced methylation, oxalate problems, and other chronic diseases.

Individuals with SULT SNPs have slower sulfation pathways already, and when phenols from the gut enter their bodies in high amounts, they slow down their phase II sulfur detoxification even more.[7] In this way, excessive phenol production from the gut bacteria can greatly impair the body's detox system, increasing sensitivity to smells, foods, chemicals, and more. The phenol connection to methylation is the idea behind the Feingold Diet for the treatment of autism and other neurological and developmental issues. The end result is that our bodies become progressively dysfunctional as phenols spill from the gut into the liver, aggravating our detoxification and methylation pathways. Even more, as adrenaline levels rise and flare our symptoms, it puts more pressure on the COMT and MAO systems, two pathways that are already genetically slowed in many people.

AROMATIC AMINO ACIDS

Aromatic amino acids that are produced by gut bacteria are necessary for proper brain and nervous system function. You've likely heard of the aromatic amino acids tyrosine, phenylalanine, and tryptophan. These are important protein precursors of dopamine, adrenaline, noradrenaline, serotonin, and melatonin neurotransmitters. These chemical messengers regulate sleep, attention, thinking, and multitudes of other critical processes. Too many or too few of these amino acids can have a large impact on our brain and our methylation cycle. You can be certain that individuals who are dealing with depression, fatigue, insomnia, anxiety, worry, panic, and pain have an imbalance in their neurotransmitters. For without optimum levels of neurotransmitters, we cannot experience optimum health, neurological or otherwise.

Although we can get these aromatic amino acids in our diet when we eat protein, the gut microbes also produce these key biomolecules. Yes, bacteria in the gut produce the amino acids we use to make our neurotransmitters, and this is one reason why the gut is often called the "second brain." This idea is supported by research that shows our gut bacteria produce significant quantities of aromatic amino acids. In a 2010 study, researchers highlighted the fact that bacteria, like plants, have a chemical pathway, called the Shikimate pathway, which allows them to produce tyrosine, phenylalanine, and tryptophan.[8] By producing the precursors to the neurotransmitters serotonin, melatonin, dopamine, and adrenaline, our gut contributes a great deal to how we think, feel, and act each day. If the gut bacteria can produce amino acids that turn into neurotransmitters, it is easy to see how our microbiome can impact our brain function.

Giving credence to this idea, researchers have now shown that diverse types of gut bacteria are capable of producing tryptophan, an essential amino acid we simply cannot live without. In a study published in 2014, researchers pointed out that gut bacteria such as Firmicutes, Proteobacteria, and E. coli can produce tryptophan, but this production is altered by use of antibiotics.[9] Let that last statement sink in for a moment: research proves antibiotics change how tryptophan is produced in our gut. Tryptophan is an essential amino acid. It is required to produce serotonin and vitamin B3. Our bodies cannot produce tryptophan, so it must come from our diet or our microbiome. Low tryptophan levels lead to a disease called pellagra, which causes diarrhea, dermatitis, dementia, and even death. Without this key amino acid, we will become deficient in vitamin B3 and be unable to produce serotonin.[10, 11] Lack of tryptophan will also lead to a loss of NAD, a powerful mitochondrial nutrient linked to muscle wasting, accelerated aging, and even cancer.[12, 13] We must keep our tryptophan, B3, and NAD levels optimized, not just for the benefit today, but for the dividends it will pay down the road (you will hear more about this important subject in chapter 10).

Given that nearly everyone reading this book has had at least one round of antibiotics in their lifetime, it would be nice to think that even a single round of antibiotics would cause no harm. And I sincerely wish I could tell you that antibiotics don't harm brain function, except that the research would disagree. Because depression is associated with low brain serotonin, and antibiotics kill bacteria that produce tryptophan, the logical question to ask would be Do antibiotics actually cause depression?

To solve the riddle of chronic disease and optimum health, we must listen to what the science is trying to tell us. The latest research confirms that antibiotic use will increase the risk of depression. In a massive study published in 2015, which included more than 1 million people, researchers showed that exposure to a single round of antibiotics increases risk of depression by 25 percent, while exposure to more than five rounds increases depression risk by more than 50 percent.[14] Now just think about all the hundreds of millions of antibiotic prescriptions used each year in the United States. What are those drugs doing to the long-term mental health of our children, our parents, and our loved ones?

If the latest research on antidepressant use is any indication, the destruction of our gut health is leading to an epidemic of depression. Due in large part to the overuse of antibiotics and destruction of our gut bugs, antidepressant use is skyrocketing! The latest research shows that 10 percent of the US population is currently taking an antidepressant, while roughly 25 percent of middle-aged women in the United States take these drugs every day.[15] In other words, a large percentage of American women who should be enjoying the prime of their lives are riddled with anxiety, depression, and other symptoms that make their daily lives a struggle. It seems like we are just trying to put a bandage on a gut-based problem by taking drugs designed to change brain chemistry. Maybe the brain isn't the problem. Maybe the gut is where we should start!

THE SHIKIMATE PATHWAY, GMOS, AND GLYPHOSATES

Before we move on, let's take one more look at the Shikimate pathway. The Shikimate pathway is the only way bacteria can produce those very important aromatic amino acids. And what happens when you eat genetically modified foods like corn, soy, wheat, and more? The Shikimate pathway gets destroyed by these life-negative chemicals. We now know that the active ingredient glyphosate destroys the Shikimate pathway in bacteria.16 Without this pathway working, the good bacteria in our bodies will tend to die off and more aggressive forms will take their place. This is the real, hidden danger of glyphosate. Not only does it act like an antibiotic in our gut, but it will alter our microbiome so that every body system, including the liver, brain, and even the methylation cycle, will suffer the effect.

Because this book focuses on how methylation and genes impact health, it is important that you understand how the environment plays a role. You've heard me say over and over again that our genes are "not our destiny, but they are our tendency." What that really means is that the environment—in our body, our homes, our food, our water, and so on—is the deciding factor of whether we experience health or disease. Genes cannot be changed except by changing the environment to improve how those genes express. And with that key concept in mind, let's turn our attention to how glyphosate, the most popular herbicide in the world, creates an environmental disaster inside our bodies. Glyphosates are powerful herbicides developed to kill weeds in croplands, and GMO foods are genetically modified to tolerate being sprayed with glyphosate herbicides such as Roundup. When we eat GMO foods grown with glyphosate herbicides, we are harming our microbiome and raising the risk of chronic diseases such as cancer and depression.

As we take a deeper look at these issues, let's again consider the work of Stephanie Seneff, PhD, an MIT researcher with more than 170 published papers under her belt. A computer science and artificial intelligence researcher by training, Seneff has applied cutting-edge data analysis techniques not only to the autism epidemic but also to the relationships between glyphosate use and cancer. What she uncovered in the data sent shockwaves through the natural health world. Analyzing data from the years 1990 to 2010, she found that glyphosate use correlated almost perfectly with the incidence and death rate for common cancers such as thyroid, liver, pancreatic, and bladder cancers. Her research shows us that the more glyphosate we use, the higher the rates of cancer and death from cancer.17 She theorizes that as healthy gut bacteria are destroyed by Roundup and other glyphosates, the intestines degenerate into a state of chronic inflammation and leaky gut, which, over time, create the perfect storm for cancer growth.

Unfortunately, glyphosate doesn't just cause gut problems, it also creates one heck of a hormone mess. Like so many toxic chemicals in our environment, glyphosate appears to mimic the activity of the female hormone estrogen. In support of this fact, researchers published a study in 2013 proving that glyphosate acts like estrogen, activating the estrogen receptor inside the cells and causing breast cancer cells to grow.18 Not only must we avoid GMO/glyphosate—grown foods because of the damage they can cause to our digestive systems, we also must limit our exposure to chemical estrogens that increase our risk of cancer in many parts of our body.

It's not only independent researchers such as Dr. Seneff who are sounding the alarm over GMO foods and the poisonous chemicals used to produce them. Even the World Health Organization has joined the conversation. In a 2015 publication from the International Agency for Research on Cancer, experts from eleven countries came together to study the data and determined that glyphosate is now a likely cause of cancer in people.[19] The WHO is a conservative organization, so when it says the active ingredient in Roundup causes cancer, we should all take notice. Adding weight to this discovery, the WHO conclusion that glyphosate is a cause of cancer was published in the prestigious medical journal The Lancet Oncology.[20] You don't need me to tell you that everyone should avoid GMO foods and eat organic as much as possible. Even though this data can save lives, it will not be shared by the companies and corporations that produce and use this toxic poison.

Regardless of our age, sex, or background, we are collectively losing the battle for our mental health because of harm to our microbiome. Not only do pharmaceutical drugs and antibiotics harm our digestion, but GMO/glyphosate-toxin-laden foods are causing serious damage as well. Each exposure to these gut toxins forces us to take a step back in our health To move our health forward and optimize our genes, we must take excellent care of our digestive system. We should always look to alternative methods such as herbs, vitamins, chiropractic care, and dietary changes before reaching for antibiotics at every little bump in the road. And eating clean, truly organic food is absolutely essential as well.

In summary, our ability to produce serotonin, dopamine, melatonin, and adrenaline depends on the availability of aromatic amino acids, many of which come from our gut. Antibiotic drugs in the food and water supply, along with GMO foods grown with glyphosate poisons, harm our gut bacteria, limiting their ability to produce these important amino acids. Methylation-related problems often involve neurological symptoms such as depression, anxiety, insomnia, worry, panic, ADD/ADHD, and more. Because the gut provides aromatic amino acids, it plays a key role in our methylation cycle and brain chemistry. When the gut bacteria cannot produce aromatic amino acids because of exposure to antibiotics, glyphosate, or other toxins, we experience depression, digestive upset, brain fog, fatigue, low energy, and other chronic health issues. In short, we experience ill health when the aromatic amino acid pathways in our gut have been compromised. It's worth it to take an effort to eat organic, avoid all unnecessary medications, and seek the advice of naturally minded doctors whenever possible. Your gut will thank you!

ALDEHYDES AND ALCOHOL

Although gut bacteria get a lot of press these days, other gut bugs need our attention as well. Among these non-bacterial gut creatures, *Candida albicans* is definitely the most important. The reason *Candida* has such a major impact on our methylation pathways has to do with the fact that this particular gut bug produces large amounts of aldehydes and alcohols.[21, 22] Yeasts such as *Candida* produce toxic molecules, which are similar in shape and function to formaldehyde, a known cancer-causing toxin used in thousands of products. As you will learn in chapter 11, aldehydes are not produced only by yeasts such as *Candida*, but they are also produced when our body breaks down the neurotransmitters serotonin, dopamine, norepinephrine, and epinephrine. It is safe to say that everyone comes into contact with aldehydes and we must all detoxify them daily.

The bigger problem with these chemicals is that they harm our DNA and our methylation-related pathways. For many years, researchers have been aware of the toxic nature of aldehydes. Studying these volatile organic chemicals gets into some pretty complicated chemistry that can make your head spin. For the purposes of our discussion, I don't need to get into too much detail. What you need to understand is that aldehydes are toxic because they can break DNA, alter the shape of proteins, speed up the aging process, and ultimately lead to cancer formation.[23] Although these yeasts and industrial toxins can potentially harm cells all over our body, the liver is the organ that bears the brunt of aldehyde toxicity.[24] The liver does so many things to keep us healthy and feeling optimum that any lack of liver function, any biochemical roadblocks that build up inside this amazing organ, can greatly impact our health. Remember that the liver is the most important organ of detoxification and it also houses a majority of our critical methylation pathways. This is why studying methylation so intensely has led me to look at the gut as a major source of methylation-related problems. With a sick, unbalanced gut environment, every component of liver function will be impaired.

Giving support to these ideas, a research team published a report in 2011 that highlighted the ways that aldehydes damage the liver. In this study, researchers looked at the aldehydes produced by smoking cigarettes— which, by the way, are chemically identical to the aldehydes produced by yeast in our gut. What they discovered was that aldehydes deplete the liver of sulfur antioxidants, leading first to autoimmune inflammation and then ultimately to cell death.[25] Clearly, you don't have to be a biochemist to know that aldehydes are a very toxic thing for the body. In fact, these chemicals are so toxic that scientists have recently shown how Alzheimer's and Parkinson's diseases are both caused in part by toxic aldehydes released during dopamine breakdown inside the brain.[26, 27] The fact that aldehydes not only injure the liver, but also impair brain function, helps us to see how chemicals from the gut can cause a wide range of health problems.

Given the link between aldehydes that are produced by Candida and the development of Parkinson's disease, we have to wonder if these two phenomena are related. And the research suggests this is a real possibility. A study published in the journal Clinical Chemistry in 2008 describes how aldehydes combine with dopamine to form salsolinol, a toxin involved in the destruction of dopamine neurons.[28] This research shows that the more aldehydes are produced, the more salsolinol is produced and the less dopamine is produced. For people dealing with challenges of Parkinson's, anything that lowers dopamine levels and increases toxins inside neurons is a threat. Although this just scratches the surface of the connection between Parkinson's and aldehydes, it is fascinating that a common gut toxin produced by a common gut bug can cause a chronic brain disease. If you ever needed evidence to look at gut health in anyone with a brain problem, here it is!

Aldehydes aren't just going to damage cells and impair the liver's detoxification system. They will also have a huge impact on the methylation cycle and the function of important genetic pathways. These volatile organic chemicals will interfere with the methylation cycle in a couple of ways. First, aldehydes from Candida are known to inhibit the methionine synthase enzyme (MTR), which is required for the recycling of homocysteine and the production of SAMe.[29, 30] This is a serious issue, because when SAMe levels drop, our methylation capacity will slow down.

Slow methylation is related to a host of health problems, from chemical sensitivity, depression, heart disease, and chronic fatigue, to autoimmune disease and cancer. The entire purpose of this book is to help you optimize your genes by supporting optimum methylation in every cell and in every organ. Slowing down methionine synthase due to high aldehyde levels will negatively impact your methylation cycle. And since many people reading this book already have untreated methylation pathway problems, any excess yeast in the gut will make methylation pathways even weaker.

The other way aldehydes interfere with methylation comes from the fact that they are derived from ethanol. In other words, when the body has a problem with yeast and aldehydes, it also has a problem with alcohol, since both chemicals are produced by Candida in large quantities. Ethanol can harm our methylation cycle in much the same way as aldehydes. Ethanol not only interferes with the absorption of vitamin B9 in the gut, but it also shuts down the MTR enzyme, leading to elevated homocysteine and poor methylation across the board.[31] And, unfortunately for our methylation cycle, aldehydes and alcohol are both broken down by the exact same enzymes that break down histamine, serotonin, dopamine, and adrenaline. When two molecules compete for the same parking space (like the phenols discussed earlier in this chapter), it slows the breakdown of those molecules, causing symptoms and upsetting the methylation pathways.

The ethanol produced by Candida leaks into the body and is converted to an aldehyde in the liver by the enzyme alcohol dehydrogenase (ADH).

Then the toxic aldehyde–whether produced directly from yeast or converted from ethanol–is further broken down into vinegar (acetic acid) by the enzyme aldehyde dehydrogenase (ALDH).[32] On the surface, this information wouldn't be earth-shattering all by itself. But like so many critical pathways in the body, both the ADH and ALDH enzymes depend on NAD/vitamin B3 to function.

As you can see in Figure 7.1, these two enzymes are a critical part of our neurotransmitter cycle. Ultimately, the more aldehydes and ethanol produced by yeasts in the gut, the more NAD is lost from the body. Since you know how important NAD is for our mitochondrial health, you can see that aldehydes will create problems for our mitochondria. Not exactly a health positive situation!

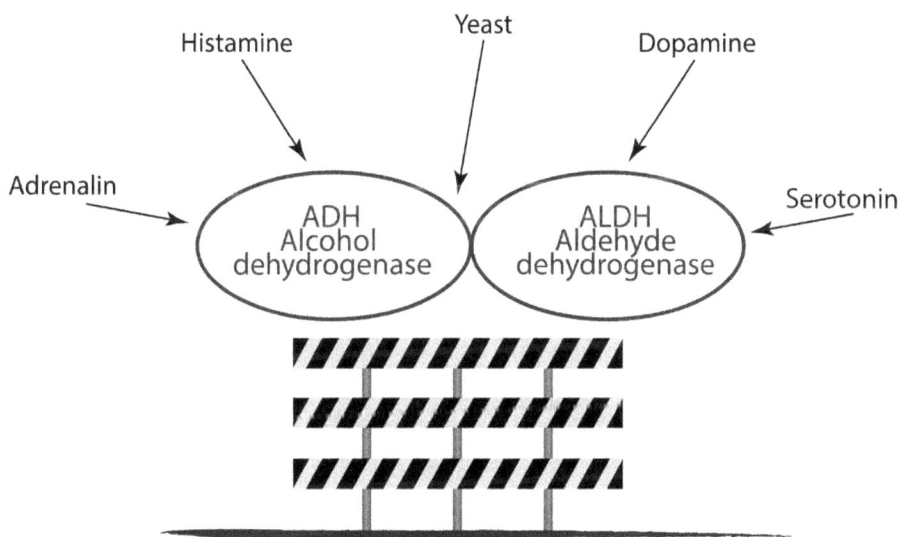

Figure 7.1 - *Dopamine, adrenaline, serotonin, Candida toxins and histamine all share the same ALDH and ADH detoxification enzymes. Slowing down the ALDH and ADH enzymes can cause increased symptoms as the body struggles to detoxify these neurotransmitters.*

I want to reiterate that we have a shared pathway between histamine and aldehydes in the liver. Many of my patients have symptoms of histamine intolerance and are unaware that their gut is the main source of their histamine problem. Histamine is actually a neurotransmitter, and when the gut is unhealthy and the liver overburdened, histamines can cause a lot of symptoms. Problems from high histamines vary widely, from headache, insomnia, diarrhea, and asthma, to low blood pressure, heart palpitations, flushing, swelling, and of course itching.[33, 34]

With a list of symptoms that long and diverse, it's easy to see how histamines could be a hidden cause of chronic, complex health issues. Just as we see with methylation problems, there is a lack of awareness in the healthcare community about histamine problems. Because of this, patients who are looking for root causes to their ill health often must do their own research to discover they have a problem with histamines. In fact, I have learned more about histamines from my patients' own experiences than anything else. If only more patients were encouraged to find their own answers, healthcare would drastically improve!

The key take-away here is to be aware that gut problems in the form of Candida infections will likely increase sensitivity to histamines because of shared detoxification pathways with dopamine, serotonin, aldehydes, and adrenaline. As you saw in Figure 7.1, alcohol and aldehydes produced by yeast put pressure on the ADH and ALDH enzymes, leaving less room for histamines to be processed and cleared from our bodies. If this happens for a short period, the body will adapt without symptoms. However, over time, the levels of histamine will rise and the levels of NAD will fall. As histamine levels rise, the body will have to use more of its methylation savings account to get rid of the histamine. The more histamine the body must deal with, the less methylation support is available for optimum brain function, digestion, energy, and repair. This is why getting rid of Candida by following the advice in this book is so essential to long-term health.

Basically, people with a Candida problem are more likely to have allergic reactions, seasonal allergies, and a low tolerance for stress. Because aldehydes, histamine, dopamine, serotonin, and adrenaline each get metabolized through the aldehyde detox pathway, excess aldehydes cause increased levels of stress hormones and neurotransmitters. This is a recipe for anxiety, worry, panic, pain, heart palpitations, sweating, insomnia, and more. When you also realize that a majority of the population also has methylation SNPs, it begins to make sense that so many people are having trouble feeling well. If we treat the gut first and then move on to fixing our other challenges, we will get much better results.

CONCLUSION

You now know that gut byproducts that increase the levels of stress hormones–phenols, aromatic amino acids, and aldehydes–will tend to cause anxiety and many other symptoms that are often found in people with methylation problems. When these SULT, COMT, ALDH, and other methylation-related pathways are blocked by gut problems, we simply lose our tolerance for stress. When stress chemicals rise inside the body, people with a gut-based methylation problem will not be able to clear these chemicals from circulation fast enough. This is a recipe for poor sleep, anxiety, worry, panic, pain, and more. But after reading this chapter, you know it doesn't have to be this way. In the protocol that follows, I share a program that can dramatically change the gut in as little as 10 days.

Clearly, the issue with gut health and methylation is a complex one, and it can have a huge impact on our health. It is a fact that our gut microbiome provides us with important nutrients that we otherwise wouldn't get in our diet. Yet it is also true that an excess of or the wrong kind of yeast and bacteria can upset our methylation cycle and make us sick. There is a reason that seasoned practitioners look first at the gut to make sure that is working properly.

If we are getting too many phenols and aldehydes, or too few aromatic amino acids from our gut into our body, we will not be able to optimize methylation by using supplements. In cases like these we must heal and balance the gut first. Healing the gut is simple, but it takes hard work. It requires effort, focus, discipline, and of course the right advice, supplements, and diet. This strategy has been the most promising in treating methylation issues that don't respond well to B-vitamin therapy. When methylation supplements give you a bad reaction, look to the gut as the origin of your methylation problem.

DR. RAKOWSKI'S 10-DAY 4R PROTOCOL

Gut dysfunction like we have discussed in this chapter can be improved in a short period of time. Dr. Robert Rakowski, a brilliant clinician, chiropractor, and healer, developed this intense protocol to help his patients restore their gut function in just 10 days. It certainly does heal the gut in a very short period of time! The only caveat I offer is this: For those with SIBO issues, who get severe bloating with probiotics and fermentable sugars, this protocol isn't your best choice. Go back to the protocol in chapter 6 and work with that one instead.

I have seen this program help individuals with long-term gut problems. Individuals who have had diarrhea for 5 years regain normal bowel movements. Individuals with 40 years of constipation begin to enjoy the relief that comes from regular, daily bowel movements. I have even seen it help those with crippling anxiety, hormone imbalance, and chronic fatigue and pain syndromes! Truly, healing the gut makes life-changing results a reality for many of our patients.

We just can't get away from the fact that healing the gut allows the body to experience greater health and well-being. And gut repair doesn't have to take months. This 10-day gut program uses high, therapeutic dosages of safe, powerful ingredients to change the gut environment quickly. The reason the program is called the "4R" program is that it removes bad bugs, repairs the gut lining, replaces digestive enzymes, and re-inoculates the gut flora with high-dose probiotics. And doing all four of these Rs at once is more powerful and effective than doing them separately.

RECOMMENDED LAB TESTING:

I recommend the Routine Blood Tests and the Organic Acid Test in appendix B for assessing the levels of phenols, aldehydes, and neurotransmitters dopamine and serotonin. Occasionally I recommend Comprehensive Stool Testing in addition, which is also found in appendix B. The stool test is useful when symptoms don't subside after this intense 10-day 4R program or when individuals are suspected of having parasites and/or inflammatory bowel issues. To make full use of the information in this book, I recommend following the instructions found in appendix A to get your own detailed genetic report.

RECOMMENDED DIET FOR THE 10-DAY 4R GUT REPAIR:

Eat only lean, organic meat and organic vegetables for 10 days. During this 10-day program, eat mono meals by eating only one food at a time. That means each time you eat, you are eating only one type of food. For example, you eat only eggs for breakfast, green beans for a mid-morning snack, grass-fed steak for lunch, asparagus for an afternoon snack, and grilled salmon for dinner. Do this for the entire 10 days. Don't be surprised if you experience some healthy weight loss on this program also! You may use MCT (Medium-chain triglyceride) oil, grass-fed cow butter, coconut oil, and avocado oil while on this protocol, since these healthy fats don't feed bad bugs one bit.

NOTE: Avoid starches, fruit, sugar, breads, cereals, etc. as these foods are fuel for the bacteria/ fungi/parasites you are trying to eliminate from your body.

RECOMMENDED SUPPLEMENT PLAN FOR THE FIRST 10 DAYS:

HCl Support – HCl stomach acid that will support the digestion and help break down your food. Take this product at the end of the meal. To find out what dose is best for you, see the HCl stomach acid instructions page.† (Nutridyn)

Pan 5X – Pancreatic enzymes that will help you break down your food. Take 1 or 2 capsules five minutes before meals/shakes/snacks. Will improve digestion and absorption of nutrients.† (Nutridyn)

NOTE: If pain or discomfort occurs when taking HCl Support, it indicates inflammation of the lining of the stomach and esophagus. To heal the stomach and esophagus, use the Gastritis Repair Protocol found in chapter 3 for at least 4 weeks before trying to reintroduce the HCl Support.

UltraBiotic Defense– 2 capsules 3 times per day with food (need two 30-capsule bottles). *Saccharomyces boulardii* is a species of bacteria that helps remove toxic yeast and fungi from sticking to the walls of the GI tract. Once yeasts and fungi are removed from the wall, your body can easily eliminate the pathogen in the stool.† (Nutridyn)

<u>UltraBiotic Daily Extra Strength</u> – 1 capsule 3 times per day away from food (need one 30-capsule bottle). High-dose probiotic 60 billion per serving to re-inoculate the colon and improve digestion.† (Nutridyn)

<u>Spectrum AR</u> – 2 softgels 3 times per day with meals. Aromatic oils that work as well as gold standard antibiotics at killing bad bugs, yet have no negative side effects. Cleanses the bowel of bacteria/viruses/yeast/parasites.† (Nutridyn)

<u>Spectrum BR</u>– 3 tablets 3 times per day with meals. Oils of berberine are very effective for removing more bacteria/viruses/yeast/parasites from the GI tract.† (Nutridyn)

<u>D3 10,000 with K2</u> – 1 softgel per day with a meal. Provides numerous benefits to the health and function of the GI tract, and patients with gut problems are chronically low in fat-soluble vitamins like D3.† (Nutridyn)

<u>L-Glutamine Powder</u> – 10-20 grams 5 times per day mixed into water. Main fuel source and nutrient source for the cells that line the GI tract. Helps to seal a leaky gut by allowing the epithelial cells to grow faster and healthier, reducing inflammation and increasing glutathione.† (Nutridyn)

RECOMMENDED DIET AND SUPPLEMENT PLAN FOR THE 30 DAYS AFTER COMPLETING THE FIRST 10 DAYS:

I recommend that my patients with gut dysbiosis issues such as those discussed in this chapter use the preceding supplements for 10 days. After the 10 days, I also recommend a follow-through period of at least 4 weeks. There is no need to continue eating in a mono meal fashion, and food may now be combined to your liking. However, it's important to continue to limit and/or avoid the high starchy foods during this 4-week period.

NOTE: You may follow the Anti-Candida Diet in appendix D for more specific instructions on which foods to avoid during the 30-day follow-through period. If you feel that an extended protocol would be beneficial to your digestive system, you may extend the timeline from 4 weeks to 8 or 12 weeks in total following the Anti-Candida Diet and taking the supplements below. Some people need a longer protocol based on their individual needs.

During the 4-week period, continue to take the exact supplements listed earlier, except reduce them in the following manner:

- Reduce the Spectrum AR to 1 softgel, 2 times per day with food.

- Reduce the Spectrum BR to 2 tablets, 2 times per day with food.

- Reduce the Glutamine Powder to 10 grams, 3 times per day.

- Reduce the UltraBiotic Defense to 1 capsule, 3 times per day with food.

- Reduce the UltraBiotic Daily Extra Strength to 1 capsule, 1 time per day away from food.

- Continue to take the Pan 5X, HCl Support, and D3 10,000 with K2.

---

†This statement has not been evaluated by the FDA. This product is not intended to diagnose, treat, cure, or prevent any disease. The information provided in this book is intended for your general knowledge only and is not a substitute for professional medical advice or treatment for specific medical conditions. You should not use this information to diagnose or treat a health problem or disease without consulting with a qualified healthcare provider. Please consult your healthcare provider with any questions or concerns you may have regarding your condition. Never disregard professional medical advice or delay in seeking it because of something you have read in this book.

REFERENCES

1. "An Interview with Steven R. Gundry, M.D., APOE, Alzheimer's, Diet, Heart," Dr. Jess Armine. Blog Talk Radio. N.p., 12 Jan. 2015. www.blogtalkradio.com/drjessarmine/2015/01/13/an-interview-with-steven-r-gundry-md-apoe-alzheimers-diet-heart.

2. Nicholson, J.K., E. Holmes, J. Kinross, et al. Host-gut microbiota metabolic interactions. *Science.* (2012) 336(6086): 1262-7.

3. Nikodejevic, B., S. Senoh, J.W. Daly, et al. Catechol-O-methyltransferase. II. A new class of inhibitors of catechol-o-methyltransferase; 3,5-dihydroxy-4-methoxybenzoic acid and related compounds. *J Pharmacol Exp Ther.* (1970) 174(1): 83-93.

4. Baldessarini, R.J., and E. Greiner. Inhibition of catechol-O-methyl transferase by catechols and polyphenols. *Biochem Pharmacol.* (1973) 22(2): 247-56.

5. Dooley, T.P. Cloning of the human phenol sulfotransferase gene family: three genes implicated in the metabolism of catecholamines, thyroid hormones and drugs. *Chem Biol Interact.* (1998) 109(1-3): 29-41.

6. Maiti, S., S. Grant, S.M. Baker, et al. Stress regulation of sulfotransferases in male rat liver. *Biochem Biophys Res Commun.* (2004) 323(1): 235-41.

7. Harris, R.M., R.H. Waring. Sulfotransferase inhibition: potential impact of diet and environmental chemicals on steroid metabolism and drug detoxification. *Curr Drug Metab.* (2008) 9(4): 269-75.

8. Tzin, V., G. Galili. New insights into the shikimate and aromatic amino acids biosynthesis pathways in plants. *Molecular Plant.* (2010) 3(6): 956-72.

9. Sharon, G., N. Garg, J. Debelius, R. Knight, et al. Specialized metabolites from the microbiome in health and disease. *Cell Metabolism.* (2014) 20(5): 719-30.

10. Hare, E.E., C.M. Loer. Function and evolution of the serotonin-synthetic bas-1 gene and other aromatic amino acid decarboxylase genes in Caenorhabditis. *BMC Evolutionary Biology.* (2004) 4(1): 24.

11. Penberthy, W.T., I. Tsunoda. The importance of NAD in multiple sclerosis. *Current Pharmaceutical Design.* (2009) 15(1): 64-99.

12. Gomes, A.P., N.L. Price, A.J. Ling, et al. Declining NAD+ induces a pseudohypoxic state disrupting nuclear-mitochondrial communication during aging. *Cell.* (2013) 155(7): 1624-38.

13. Mendelsohn, A.R., J.W. Larrick. Partial reversal of skeletal muscle aging by restoration of normal NAD+ levels. *Rejuvenation Research.* (2014) 17(1): 62-9.

14. Lurie, I., Y.X. Yang, K. Haynes, et al. Antibiotic exposure and the risk for depression, anxiety, or psychosis: a nested case-control study. *The Journal of Clinical Psychiatry.* (2015) 76(11): 1522.

15. Calderone, J. The Rise of All-Purpose Antidepressants. *Scientific American* website. www.scientificamerican.com/article/the-rise-of-all-purpose-antidepressants/. (2014). Accessed January 26, 2017.

16. Amrhein, N., B. Deus, P. Gehrke, et al. The site of the inhibition of the shikimate pathway by glyphosate II. Interference of glyphosate with chorismate formation in vivo and in vitro. *Plant Physiology*. (1980) 66(5): 830-4.

17. Samsel, A., S. Seneff. Glyphosate, pathways to modern diseases IV: cancer and related pathologies. *J. Biol. Phys. Chem.* (2015) 15: 121-59.

18. Thongprakaisang, S., A. Thiantanawat, N. Rangkadilok, et al. Glyphosate induces human breast cancer cells growth via estrogen receptors. *Food Chem Toxicol.* (2013) 59: 129-36.

19. International Agency for Research on Cancer, World Health Organization website. IARC monographs volume 112: evaluation of five organophosphate insecticides and herbicides. www.iarc.fr/en/media-centre/iarcnews/pdf/MonographVolume112.pdf. (2015). Accessed January 26, 2017.

20. Guyton, K.Z., D. Loomis, Y. Grosse, et al. Carcinogenicity of tetrachlorvinphos, parathion, malathion, diazinon, and glyphosate. *Lancet Oncol.* (2015) 16(5): 490-1.

21. Gainza-Cirauqui, M.L., M.T. Nieminen, L. Novak Frazer, et al. Production of carcinogenic acetaldehyde by *Candida albicans* from patients with potentially malignant oral mucosal disorders. *Journal of Oral Pathology & Medicine*. (2013) 42(3): 243-9.

22. Marttila, E., P. Bowyer, D. Sanglard, et al. Fermentative 2-carbon metabolism produces carcinogenic levels of acetaldehyde in *Candida albicans*. *Molecular Oral Microbiology*. (2013) 28(4): 281-91.

23. O'Brien, P.J., A.G. Siraki, N. Shangari. Aldehyde sources, metabolism, molecular toxicity mechanisms, and possible effects on human health. *Critical Reviews in Toxicology*. (2005) 35(7): 609-62.

24. Cho, I., M.J. Blaser. The human microbiome: at the interface of health and disease. *Nature Reviews Genetics*. (2012) 13(4): 260-70.

25. Yao, H., I. Rahman. Current concepts on oxidative/carbonyl stress, inflammation and epigenetics in pathogenesis of chronic obstructive pulmonary disease. *Toxicology and Applied Pharmacology*. (2011) 254(2): 72-85.

26. Burke, W.J., S.W. Li, C.A. Schmitt, P. Xia, et al. Accumulation of 3,4-dihydroxyphenylglycolaldehyde, the neurotoxic monoamine oxidase A metabolite of norepinephrine, in locus ceruleus cell bodies in Alzheimer's disease: mechanism of neuron death. *Brain Research*. (1999) 816(2): 633-7.

27. Marchitti, S.A., R.A. Deitrich, V. Vasiliou. Neurotoxicity and metabolism of the catecholamine-derived 3, 4-dihydroxyphenylacetaldehyde and 3, 4-dihydroxyphenylglycolaldehyde: the role of aldehyde dehydrogenase. *Pharmacological Reviews*. (2007) 59(2): 125-50.

28. Zhu, W., D. Wang, J. Zheng, et al. Effect of (R)-salsolinol and N-methyl-(R)-salsolinol on the balance impairment between dopamine and acetylcholine in rat brain: involvement in pathogenesis of Parkinson disease. *Clinical Chemistry.* (2008) 54(4): 705-12.

29. Waly, M.I., K.K. Kharbanda, R.C. Deth. Ethanol Lowers Glutathione in Rat Liver and Brain and Inhibits Methionine Synthase in a Cobalamin-Dependent Manner. *Alcoholism: Clinical and Experimental Research.* (2011) 35(2): 277-83.

30. Barak, A.J., H.C. Beckenhauer, D.J. Tuma. Methionine synthase: a possible prime site of the ethanolic lesion in liver. *Alcohol.* (2002) 26(2): 65-7.

31. Zakhari, S. Alcohol metabolism and epigenetics changes. *Alcohol Res.* (2013) 35(1): 6-16.

32. Chen, C.H., J.C. Ferreira, E.R. Gross, et al. Targeting aldehyde dehydrogenase 2: new therapeutic opportunities. *Physiological Reviews.* (2014) 94(1): 1-34.

33. Smolinska, S., M. Jutel, R. Crameri, et al. Histamine and gut mucosal immune regulation. *Allergy.* (2014) 69(3): 273-81.

34. Thurmond, R.L., E.W. Gelfand, P.J. Dunford. The role of histamine H1 and H4 receptors in allergic inflammation: the search for new antihistamines. *Nature Reviews Drug Discovery.* (2008) 7(1): 41-53.

8.

METHYLATION AND THE
STRESS-GUT CONNECTION

It's not stress that kills us, it is our reaction to it.

—Hans Selye

Now that you have seen how gut problems create serious issues with methylation, mood, and mitochondria, another part of the gut story must be told. No understanding of gut health would be complete without looking at how stress impacts the digestive system. As you might imagine, stress has an enormous impact on *who* and *what* lives in our gut.

Over and over again in my practice, people tell me they never had a digestion issue or gut problem before they got sick. My patients struggle to understand why they developed a gut problem when their main complaint was in some other part of their body—brain, liver, kidneys, muscles, bones, and so on. I have wondered the same thing, too: Why do people who initially get sick from chronic fatigue, severe whiplash, or adrenal fatigue end up with gut issues? It didn't make sense right away, until I learned the science I am sharing with you in this chapter.

Getting sick is like getting stuck on a dirt road in the mud. The more you spin your tires unsuccessfully, the more stuck you become. After a while, if you keep spinning your tires, you end up digging a sizeable hole in the road that swallows your tire. Now, instead of just getting stuck in the mud, you've created a hole you have to dig out of as well. This is similar to what happens to individuals who experience a major health crash.

People who endure unexpected loss, divorce, bankruptcy, emotional and physical abuse or neglect, and other traumas may not have started with a gut problem. When driving down the muddy road of life, they didn't get stuck in a hole. They dug the hole trying to get unstuck, which created two problems to deal with. In a similar way, people who experience profound stress in life also dig themselves a proverbial hole, except in almost every case this "hole" ends up being a gut problem they didn't know they had.

They didn't enter the crisis with a digestive problem, and perhaps they had great digestion for years. But once they enter and move through the crisis, all the stress hormones and adrenaline that are released through the process absolutely and without question impact the health of the digestive tract.

Stress impacts our health in ways we are just now beginning to understand. And how the digestive system is impacted by stress is the focus of exciting new research that sheds light on many questions regarding health and methylation.

THE STRESS-GUT SCENARIO

Stress in our lives creates stress in our gut. That is a known and predictable fact of science. What is less clear, and what is the focus of this chapter, is just how those effects of stress create such a mess of our digestive system. As you

SNPs of Concern

The fact is that certain genes make us more susceptible to stress. They don't cause our stress, but they do amplify the negative effects of stress. In my opinion, the most important genes for stress are:

- *ACE – Angiotensin Converting Enzyme*
- *COMT – Catechol-O-Methyl-Transferase*
- *GAD – Glutamic Acid Decarboxylase*
- *MAO – Monoamine Oxidase*
- *MTHFR – Methyl-Tetra-Hydro-Folate-Reductase*

When we are stressed we release high levels of adrenaline (aka epinephrine or catecholamines) and this is where the stress symptoms come from. Stress chemicals such as adrenaline, dopamine, and norepinephrine often cause rapid heartbeat, sweating, panic attacks, trembling, anxiety, dizziness, etc. Being dopamine or catecholamine dominant leaves you feeling wired and tired. It causes you to feel like you just had 10 cups of coffee but all you want in the world is to relax and rest – the brain is overactivated yet fatigued at the same time.

will soon learn, stress in any form—whether physical, mental, or chemical—causes the release of adrenaline directly into the gut.

If you want to know how stress is impacting someone's life, just ask them how their digestion is working. Chances are that if they have a problem handling stress, they will have problems with their digestion—and their brain, too! Intense stress triggers the release of high levels of catecholamines directly into the bloodstream and the gut. Everyone has experienced the effect of these powerful, mind-altering stress chemicals. However, some people are exquisitely sensitive to these chemicals and can get ill from the side effects of too much adrenaline. As I have shown throughout this book, those with MAO, COMT, ACE, GAD, and MTHFR SNPs have a more difficult time handling these adrenaline molecules.

Difficulty handling stress often shows the following symptoms:

- Bloating
- Pain
- Gas
- Diarrhea
- Constipation
- Irritable bowel
- Anxiety
- Insomnia
- Depression
- Rage
- Panic attacks
- Indigestion
- Acid reflux

- And much more...

The symptoms on this list are common in nearly every patient we work with. Whether we are working over the phone, via Skype, or in person at our Boise clinic, we see these symptoms every day. Patients come from all walks of life and different backgrounds, with a wide array of different challenges. Despite the wide variety of our amazing patients, they share a common thread: they experience a high degree of stress, and as a result, they develop some problematic gut issues. From my experience, the rare individual is not the person with a gut problem; the rare individual is the person without one.

THE LEAKY GUT AND STRESS CONNECTION

Without a doubt, one of the worst stress-gut problems Americans suffer from is leaky gut, in which undigested food, bacteria, parasites, toxins, and other things inside our digestive tract are able to leak through the gut lining and into the body. This isn't great for our health; it describes a gut lining that isn't doing its job. Like good fences make good neighbors, our gut lining keeps our neighbors—the rest of the body and immune system—safe from all the bugs, food, and other stuff floating through the gut. The last thing we want is the immune system to get triggered and start attacking the body because the gut lining isn't working. This can lead to fatigue, aches, pains, inflammation, and autoimmune disease.

Luckily, there is a growing awareness that healthy digestion is part of a healthy lifestyle, and more and more people who aren't feeling well are beginning to realize that they are sick because of their gut. Even yogurt commercials are educating viewers about the fact that 70 percent of our immune system lives inside the wall of the gut.

Ultimately, the goal with gut health is to optimize the function of the GI tract. There are multiple ways to optimize gut function, which is why I've focused on this issue throughout this book (and you'll find some great info on the brain and neurotransmitters waiting for you in the final chapters). Remember that the gut performs several important roles when functioning properly. First, it allows nutrients to enter the body, which nourishes cells and allows life to continue. Second, it helps detoxify the body of waste products, which are removed from the liver via the gallbladder into the bile. And, third, the gut helps the immune system to function properly.

Most people know about the first two roles, but the third role is just as important. People with a leaky and stressed-out gut will have issues with all three of those aspects, but immune system issues are the biggest. Because the immune system can affect and access all areas of our body, leaky gut irritates not just our gut but literally the entire body.

If you counted up all the lymph nodes in the body, about 70 percent of them would be found inside special lymphatic masses called Peyer's patches, which are also known as gut-associated lymphatic tissue (or GALT). Peyer's patches function as the white-blood-cell headquarters, keeping our gut working properly. They are necessary to keep our gut from leaking toxic substances into the body. They do this mainly by producing Secretory Immunoglobulin A (SIgA), which may be familiar to you because it is an immunoglobulin like IgG or IgE and is commonly tested by stool testing from your functional medicine doctor.

SIgA is more than just a simple immunoglobulin, however. It is the glue that maintains the integrity of the gut wall. It acts like a barbed wire fence in the gut to keep bacteria and antigens that come from our diet from leaking into the body.[1] With good SIgA levels, the body is much less likely to have leaky gut and gut-brain inflammation. When SIgA levels drop, as happens when we experience chronic stress, the gut lining becomes stressed and starts to get leaky.

Chronic stress involves elevations of cortisol, and cortisol plays a big role in disturbing our sleep, immune system, and especially digestion. High stress that elevates cortisol can come from chronic illness, athletic overtraining, restrictive and imbalanced diets, and psychological stressors at home or work. Yet, regardless of what is causing the cortisol to rise, the effect on the gut is always the same.

Cortisol and adrenaline decrease the production of SIgA, which weakens our mucosal defenses, leading to leaky gut symptoms.[2] In addition, chronic stress forces blood into our muscles and away from our gut wall, leading to even more gut-barrier dysfunction. This blood-flow problem can become so bad that ulcers may develop in the stomach and areas of the intestine may be damaged by low oxygen.[3] If that weren't enough, stress also changes how blood flows to the skin. We know that the same stress hormones that reduce blood-flow to the gut also reduce blood circulation to the skin.[4] This can result in Raynaud's syndrome or other chronic blood-flow problems that are all side effects of excess cortisol and adrenaline in the system.

The take-home message here is that stress hurts our gut and our digestion. We all know that by now. And this is made worse with SNPs for IgA. People with IgA genes will be the first to feel digestive upset, pain, and discomfort in response to stress. In these individuals, it is important to keep excess stress under control so the gut can do its job. Regardless of your genes, though, lowering stress and managing cortisol levels appropriately will greatly improve your digestion. Leaky gut is a big deal, and people with high cortisol, high stress, and the related SNPs (MAO, COMT, IgA, ACE, and so on) need to be extra diligent and careful.

STRESS HORMONES AND GUT BUGS

I've listed the most important genes that influence our level of stress and catecholamines. But I haven't mentioned yet how stress hormones and neurotransmitters impact gut bacteria. Regardless of your genes, when you experience stress of any kind, it will drastically impact the health of your gut through interaction with the bacteria themselves. And, remember, the cause of the stress doesn't matter because the reaction is always the same.

Whether we are dealing with low blood sugar, food allergies, a stressful work environment, marital problems, or a sick loved one, the body's stress reaction is identical. No matter the cause of the stress, the body always reacts in a predetermined and predictable manner. This is very important to keep in mind as we explore how stress impacts our gut and our genes.

Based on the latest research, it is clear that healthy digestion is almost impossible during periods of stress. In a study published in 2008 looking at how stress impacts the microbiome, researchers highlighted the fact that about 50 percent of the norepinephrine released in the body goes straight into our gut.[5] In other words, every single human on Earth releases adrenaline into the gut each time the sympathetic nervous system is activated, no matter what SNPs they have!

This is a huge deal, since it means that the gut bacteria are getting doused with adrenaline at the same time as our heart, brain, liver, muscle, and other tissues. Because we release half of our adrenaline into the gut lumen (inside space of the gut), the bacteria living there can use these stress signals to their advantage. The same 2008 study also demonstrated that the bugs in our digestive tracts have receptors on their bodies that tell them when we are stressed. And when these bugs sense that we are stressed, they begin to change in startling ways.

To illustrate this point, the scientists performed an experiment comparing the growth rate of E. coli with and without the presence of catecholamines. The researchers attempted to reproduce the conditions in the gut that occur when a person experiences fight or flight, which for many is a daily routine. They added catecholamine stress hormones dopamine, epinephrine, and norepinephrine to petri dishes with a sample of E. coli. They then compared the growth of these stress-stimulated E. coli strains against identical strains grown in a petri dish without any stress hormones. The researchers discovered that under the influence of catecholamine stress hormones, the E. coli grew up to up to 990,000 percent more versus the bacteria without catecholamine exposure.[5] Yes, that is a massive increase! And it's all due to the effects of adrenaline, as shown in Figure 8.1.

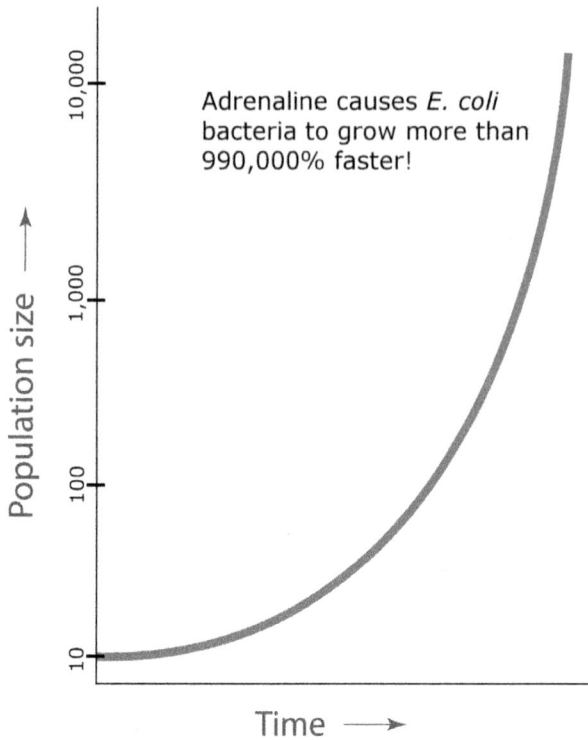

Figure 8.1 - *Adrenaline causes E. coli to grow more than 990,000 percent faster.*

A study from 2002 published in the journal *Shock* confirms these findings. The authors showed that catecholamines released after a traumatic event, such as a motor vehicle accident or surgery, caused *E. coli* to grow significantly faster.[6] They were careful to mention that the type of *E. coli* they studied was not an aggressive strain, meaning that even healthy bacteria will grow rapidly in the presence of adrenaline/epinephrine. This is just more proof that when our bodies are under stress, bacteria grow rapidly and can potentially make us sick. Thus, excess stress is likely a contributor to SIBO, since stress promotes rapid growth of gut bugs.

And it's not just *E. coli* that responds to stress by growing rapidly. We now know that many different species of bacteria respond aggressively when they come into contact with adrenaline released from our bodies. In a 2010 study published in *Infectious Immunology*, the authors showed that mice infected with *Citrobacter rodentium* that experienced severe stress showed a major change in their gut bacteria.[7] In another 2010 study from the same journal, researchers demonstrated that norepinephrine caused rapid growth in a Salmonella species that is found in our digestive tracts.[8] These studies highlight how our own gut bacteria become quite imbalanced during periods of stress, and this ultimately makes us more likely to develop a gut infection. The studies' authors suggest that when the delicate balance of the gut is disturbed, the bad bugs are more likely to take advantage, grow, and cause our health to suffer. And I for one couldn't agree more with this idea, because I routinely see this phenomenon at play in my practice.

The bugs that have so much to do with our health and well-being are constantly watching for signs that we may be under stress. The problem is that when these bacteria get a signal that we are under stress, they begin to grow rapidly and become more aggressive. The adrenaline released into the gut is a signal that the host is under duress, and from a bacteria's point of view, it is a good time to grow the family. The bugs in our gut are always looking for signals about the health of the host. When adrenaline is released, the body is basically saying to the bacteria, "Hey, go ahead and multiply! I'm busy fighting for my life (real or imagined) so my immune system won't be able to attack very well right now." Get the picture?

Our clinic attracts many chronically ill patients who have often been through severe, life-changing stresses, and they've also developed severe gut problems. These patients often don't understand why they aren't getting better. Since the stressor is behind them, why aren't they back to feeling their best? The answer lies in realizing that although the stress was the triggering factor, it was the digestive system that suffered most while they were in the state of fight or flight. So even though the stress is behind them, the gut still has to be repaired! This is so common for my patients that I have to remind new patients on multiple occasions that their genetic problems can't be addressed until their gut health is restored. You'll hear that from me over and over again throughout this book. Genes are not your destiny, but your digestion might be!

STRESS, IRON, BACTERIA

If the rapid bacterial growth caused by adrenaline isn't enough, adrenaline also gives the bacteria access to our iron supplies. Adrenaline and other catecholamines help bacteria to tear iron off of transport proteins. Because iron is needed for bacteria to grow, our body makes sure that bacteria can't easily access our iron reserves. We put our iron on "armored trucks," called lactoferrin and transferrin—this way, only we get to use it—and the iron is delivered where we want it. In a study published in 2010, researchers investigated how bacteria might rob us of our iron when we are under stress. They discovered that catecholamines bind tightly to lactoferrin and transferrin, which dislodges the iron, making it available for bacteria to eat and grow.[9] Even before this study connected the dots between stress, iron, and bacterial growth, researchers had shown that catecholamines cause an increase in free iron, which then becomes available for bacterial growth.[10]

The moral of the story is that when adrenaline is dumped into the gut, it allows the bad bugs to hijack the iron off the lactoferrin and transferrin armored trucks. A virtual robbery happening in our gut! This may cause chronic anemia and a host of other related problems in the brain and elsewhere. If the body loses iron it needs and bad bugs use it to grow, it's a sure bet that the gut and our brain won't be feeling optimally healthy. This is one of the main reasons why people who are chronically under physical or emotional stress develop problems such as SIBO, *Candida*, and leaky gut.

STRESS AND LEAKY GUT, ENDOTOXIN SNOWBALL EFFECT

By now it is easy for you to see how the stress in our lives leads to imbalances of the bacteria in our gut. And if you think all this adrenaline may lead to leaky gut, you are right! Not only does the adrenaline from stress feed bad bacteria, but it also compromises the lining of our intestines. Leaky gut is a subject that has gained more and more attention recently, even in traditional medicine, which is finally connecting the dots between the gut and the immune system. For the purpose of this discussion, you need to understand how stress contributes to the leaky gut problem.

In a 2015 study published in the journal *Frontiers in Immunology*, researchers compiled evidence showing that adrenaline causes holes to form in the gut wall, bacteria to leak into our bodies, and inflammation to increase across the board.[11] When we get stressed, a flood of dead bacteria enters through the gut and into the bloodstream. We call these toxic dead bacteria lipopolysaccharides, or LPS. When toxic bacteria leak into the bodies through the gut, it increases inflammation, which increases depression (more on this in chapter 10).[12] For a simple visual of this whole gut-brain concept, check out Figure 8.2.

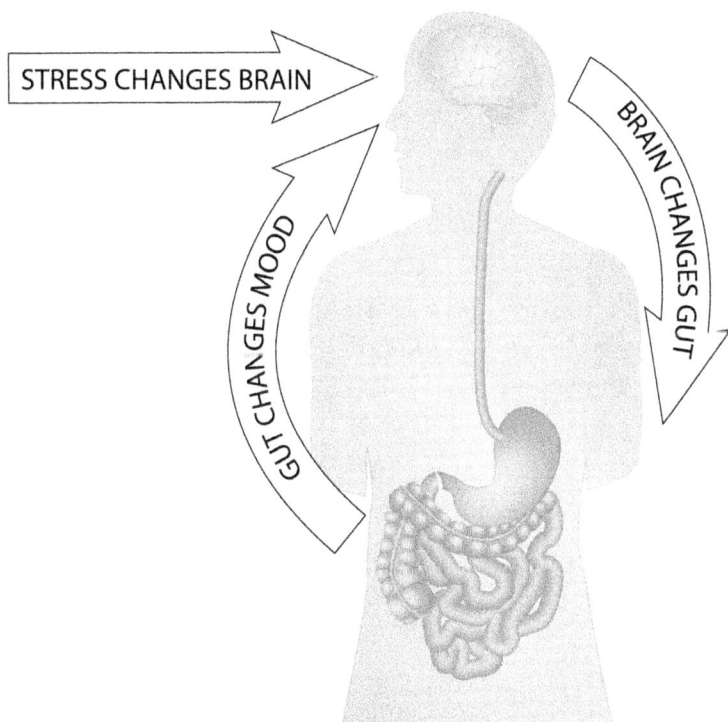

Figure 8.2 – *Stress changes our brain, then the brain changes the gut, and finally the gut changes our mood. A simple, yet powerful, process!*

When the gut is irritated and inflamed, as it is when adrenaline wreaks havoc on our gut bugs and gut lining, the number of healthy bacteria in our gut decline. Studies have proven that healthy gut bacteria boost our brain function, mood, and behavior. Not only do probiotics increase GABA, our only calming neurotransmitter, but they also communicate directly with our brain via the vagus nerve, leading to decreased anxiety, lower pain, less depression, and less brain fog.[13, 14, 15] If this is the healing power of probiotics, then imagine how difficult it is for people with bad bacteria in their gut to enjoy health and well-being. It is impossible to be healthy, impossible to optimize your genes, without first optimizing your gut!

Each and every time our sympathetic nervous system—the adrenaline-and cortisol-releasing part of our nervous system—becomes activated, we suffer a serious case of leaky gut and bacterial chaos. In modern society, people are dealing with so much stress that their digestion is barely working at all. To overcome this, we can begin to learn how stress is hurting us and make the powerful changes necessary to lower our stress, improve our digestion, and optimize our genes.

CONCLUSION

Bacteria live in our bodies in a give-and-take situation. They take up residence in our gut (mostly) and they send out chemical signals that either help us experience health or chronically poison us. And it's easy to get mad at these gut bugs and want them gone. I'm all for that, but the question of why they grew there in the first place needs to be addressed. We all have Candida and E. coli and other pathogens in our gut. They belong there as part of the normal gut environment. The problem arises, however, when the environment changes, and the gut bacteria change along with it. This is the key point to understand: our gut health and the bugs living there reflect the environment of the gut itself.

Gut bacteria can be both "good" and "bad." They can change their behavior based on signals from the host (us). We now know that half our adrenaline enters the gut each time we experience stress. This wouldn't be a big deal unless the "bad" gut bacteria could use this catecholamine neurotransmitter to their advantage—and, unfortunately, they are able to do that. In a sick twist of fate, or biochemistry (take your pick), the gut bacteria are always listening for signals from the host.

If we send them stress signals, they will take that opportunity to increase and grow, steal our iron, and become more aggressive. It's a give-and-take, remember. If we give the gut signals that life is full of stress, fear, doom, and other negative emotions, we are literally giving the signal for the bacteria in our gut to grow rapidly. And rapidly growing gut bacteria such as E. coli or Salmonella often make us sick.

The solution to all this is to limit your exposure to stress and do the simple, fundamental things every day that prevent your body from going into fight or flight. Eat every 2 or 3 hours, eat low glycemic foods, pray or meditate, spend time doing things that bring you joy, avoid things that bring you pain or sadness, and sleep at least 8 hours each night. By lowering stress, you lower adrenaline. Less adrenaline means less fuel for bad bugs to grow. In everything we do each day, our job is to use as little adrenaline as possible, for we should be saving this powerful chemical for when we really need it instead of squeezing the lemon dry each day to the detriment of our digestion, our brain, and our health. By reducing your stress and taking the right supplements at the right time, you'll truly begin to change your gut, your genes, and your life.

STRESS GUT PROTOCOL

Fixing the stress-gut issues discussed in this chapter takes a two-pronged approach: you need tools to help your body do a better job of dealing with stress, and you need to make sure your gut is healthy. For those of you who have been dealing with gut problems that are triggered by stress, you have probably developed a nasty imbalance of bacteria and yeast. Your first order of business is to go back to chapters 4, 5, 6, and 7 and make sure you follow the appropriate protocols to improve your gut health. Those protocols are necessary to undertake before you get to work healing the gut. In other words, if you treat the stress issues without taking time to heal the gut, your results will be less than optimum. I highly recommend you follow the appropriate gut protocol(s) from those chapters—this will help you fix your stress issues a lot faster.

We have all heard of using adrenal support, herbs, vitamins, minerals, adaptogens, etc., to help lessen the effects of stress on our bodies. These tools are great, and we use them with our patients every day. However, the point is to make sure you select the right tool for your body. Some people experience high cortisol and high adrenaline, while others experience low cortisol plus low adrenaline. Adrenal fatigue and chronic stress is a bell-curve like everything else in our bodies. We need to know if we are high or low before we can select the right tool.

This is a simple protocol, but it will get you started. Read the symptoms associated with each category and make your selection based on the best fit. The right adrenal support will make an almost immediate difference in your energy, sleep, focus, and mood.

RECOMMENDED LAB TESTING:

I recommend the Routine Blood Tests and the DUTCH hormone test in appendix B for assessing how effects of stress are impacting your body's metabolic and hormonal pathways. To make full use of the information in this book, I recommend following the instructions found in appendix A to get your own detailed genetic report.

HIGH-CORTISOL / HIGH-STRESS PROTOCOL:

For overactive adrenal glands that leave you feeling wired and worried:

> Stress Essentials Serenity – 2 capsules 2 times per day. Powerful blend of Chinese herbs that are demonstrated to calm and sooth excessive tension, especially on the heart.† (Nutridyn)

> Stress Essentials Calm – 2 capsules 1-2 times per day. Contains L-theanine and GABA to help reduce anxiety and activate GABA receptors inside the brain.† (Nutridyn)

For overactive adrenal glands in the evening that make it hard to fall asleep, turn off your mind:

<u>Cortisol Pro</u> - 1 capsule every hour starting 4 or 5 hours before bed time. Powerful blend of nutrients, herbs and extracts that work together to lower the output of cortisol from the adrenal glands, improving length, depth and quality of sleep.† (Nutridyn)

LOW-CORTISOL PROTOCOL:

For fatigued adrenal glands with low testosterone and/or low DHEA levels:

<u>Stress Essentials Adrenal Renew</u> - 2 capsules with breakfast and 2 capsules with lunch. Bovine adrenal extract to improve adrenal function and sex hormone levels.† (Nutridyn)

<u>Liposomal DHEA</u> - 1 to 6 doses per day. Dissolve in the mouth for 20 seconds and then swallow. Liposomal DHEA helps combat low sex hormone levels and improve resistance to stress and immune health.† (Nutridyn)

For symptoms of adrenal fatigue including dizziness, salt craving, and low blood sugar:

<u>Stress Essentials Licorice Complex</u>- 1 to 4 capsules per day. Herbal support that will increase cortisol naturally and improve blood flow; helps prevent dizziness and increases tolerance to stress.† (Nutridyn)

<u>Stress Essentials Adrenal B1B6</u> - 1 tablet with breakfast and 1 tablet at lunch. High doses of B1 and B6 and vitamin C necessary to produce Coenzyme A (CoA), a key energy molecule; also helps with adrenal hormones and supports healthy response to stress and low blood sugar.† (Nutridyn)

For symptoms of chronic stress that leave you feeling fatigued and tired:

<u>Stress Essentials Balance</u>- 2 capsules 2 times per day. Designed to build resilience and enhance stamina in individuals who are feeling weak and fatigued due to stress.† (Nutridyn)

REFERENCES

1. Brandzaeg, P. Induction of secretory immunity and memory at mucosal surfaces. *Vaccine.* (2007) 25(30): 5467-84.

2. Martínez-Carrillo, B.E., M. Godinez-Victoria, A. Jarillo-Luna, R. Oros-Pantoja, et al. Repeated restraint stress reduces the number of IgA-producing cells in Peyer's patches. *Neuroimmunomodulation.* (2011) 18(3): 131-41.

3. Bailey, R.W., G.B. Bulkley, S.R. Hamilton, et al. The fundamental hemodynamic mechanism underlying gastric "stress ulceration" in cardiogenic shock. *Ann Surg.* (1987) 205(6): 597-612.

4. Yamamoto, J., M. Nakai, T. Natsume. Cardiovascular responses to acute stress in young-to-old spontaneously hypertensive rats. *Hypertension.* (1987) 9(4): 362-70.

5. Freestone, P.P., S.M. Sandrini, R.D. Haigh, M. Lyte. Microbial endocrinology: how stress influences susceptibility to infection. *Trends Microbiol.* (2008) 16(2): 55-64.

6. Freestone, P.P., P.H. Williams, R.D. Haigh, et al. Growth stimulation of intestinal commensal *Escherichia coli* by catecholamines: a possible contributory factor in trauma-induced sepsis. *Shock.* (2002) 18(5): 465-70.

7. Bailey, M.T., S.E. Dowd, N.M. Parry, et al. Stressor exposure disrupts commensal microbial populations in the intestines and leads to increased colonization by *Citrobacter rodentium*. *Infect Immun.* (2010) 78(4): 1509-19.

8. Pullinger, G.D., S.C. Carnell, F.F. Sharaff, et al. Norepinephrine augments *Salmonella enterica*-induced enteritis in a manner associated with increased net replication but independent of the putative adrenergic sensor kinases QseC and QseE. *Infect Immun.* (2010) 78(1): 372-80.

9. Sandrini, S.M., R. Shergill, J. Woodward, et al. Elucidation of the mechanism by which catecholamine stress hormones liberate iron from the innate immune defense proteins transferrin and lactoferrin. *J Bacteriol.* (2010) 192(2): 587-94.

10. Monteiro, H.P., C.C. Winterbourn. 6-Hydroxydopamine releases iron from ferritin and promotes ferritin-dependent lipid peroxidation. *Biochem Pharmacol.* (1989) 38(23): 4177-82.

11. de Punder, K., L. Pruimboom. Stress induces endotoxemia and low-grade inflammation by

---

increasing barrier permeability. *Front Immunol*. (2015) 6: 223.

12. Ait-Belgnaoui, A., H. Durand, C. Cartier, et al. Prevention of gut leakiness by a probiotic treatment leads to attenuated HPA response to an acute psychological stress in rats. *Psychoneuroendocrinology*. (2012) 37(11): 1885–95.

13. Cryan, J.F., T.B. Dinan. Mind-altering microorganisms: the impact of the gut microbiota on brain and behaviour. *Nat Rev Neurosci*. (2012) 13(10): 701–12.

14. Savignac, H.M., G. Cornoa, H. Mille, et al. Prebiotic feeding elevates central brain derived neurotrophic factor, N-methyl-D-aspartate receptor subunits and D-serine. *Neurochem Int*. (2013) 63(8): 756–64.

15. Bravo, J.A., P. Forsythe, M.V. Chew, et al. Ingestion of Lactobacillus strain regulates emotional behavior and central GABA receptor expression in a mouse via the vagus nerve. *Proc Natl Acad Sci USA*. (2011) 108(38): 16050– 16055.

9

———

BLOOD SUGAR, METHYLATION, AND DEPRESSION

However beautiful the strategy, you should
occasionally look at the results.

—Benjamin Franklin

The desire to understand why we are sick is a powerful force; it can push us to investigate very complicated subjects. Subjects that we have already covered, such as methylation, oxalates, SIBO, and more, are fertile ground for finding answers to complex, chronic health problems. When we start looking for the keys to unlock the body's real genius to create lasting health, we often find ourselves studying some of the most complicated processes in the body. We may perform testing to look at our hormones and digestive system. We may study our inherited genetic imbalances and look for hidden infections that could be making us sick. These are all very good strategies. The logic is usually that the sicker we are, the more chronic our health problems, and the more complicated the solution must be. This is a common thought process in many who are seeking to optimize their genes and change their life.

But I must caution you against thinking that all complex problems have complex answers. Because of the beauty of how the body operates and organizes itself, simple problems are often responsible for creating complex health issues. And few simple problems are more notorious for messing with our health than low blood sugar.

As you have seen throughout this book, the simple parts are critical. We know that all complex systems such as epigenetics are built out of simple parts. The fascinating thing about studying genes and epigenetics is that it doesn't diminish the simple parts. In fact, it amplifies them! This is especially true when we turn our attention to low blood sugar, depression, and methylation.

In the next two chapters, we will journey into the simple causes of and cures for depression. We will unravel this mysterious problem by learning about how our blood sugar and insulin control how much serotonin and dopamine we produce. We will get to know the amino acid tryptophan and discover how hard it is to keep our levels in an optimum range. We will even look at genes that influence our tryptophan levels in both the gut and the brain.

In the next chapter, we will dive deeper and talk about what happens after tryptophan enters our brain. Along the way, you will learn much about the causes of depression. You will see the connections between blood sugar, insulin, tryptophan, and serotonin and learn how to balance their levels naturally.

DEPRESSION IS NOT A DRUG DEFICIENCY

I often remind my patients that we aren't depressed because of a drug deficiency. When we become depressed, it is a symptom of a brain not working properly. In fact, modern neurology and brain research now refer to depression as simply a brain that is not able to activate fast enough. Functional MRI studies comparing healthy brain scans to depressed brain scans have found that, compared to the brains of people without depression, the brains of people with depression are unable to activate fast enough.[1] Based on that information, we can say that depression is defined as a slowed down neurological system. The speed of the brain and nervous system is depressed, thus making us *feel* depressed.

I like to point out this definition of depression because we still live in a world where depression is a bit of a stigma and not everyone is willing to talk about it. Once we realize that depression is nothing more than a slowed down brain, we can start to look for and treat the root causes. Once we fix the root causes of our slowed and depressed brain, we can learn what steps are necessary to speed up the brain. And nothing is more effective at speeding up our brain than the methylation cycle and MTHFR-related genetic pathways.

Sharon contacted my office because she had seen our YouTube videos about gut health, methylation, and optimizing genes. She was in a decades-long battle with depression that didn't let up no matter what. Sharon already was doing many healthy things–yoga, organic eating, saunas, and more. She was very confused about why her depression wouldn't lift and why she had required medication for her neurotransmitters year after year. During our first consultation, I explained to her that despite her best efforts and the effects of her medication, she simply didn't have enough serotonin in her brain. I shared with her how her MTHFR genes and related genetic imbalances were making it difficult for her body to provide the raw material her brain needed. We also discussed how the gut supports brain function and that any imbalances of yeast or bacteria will be obstacles to her recovery. We ended that conversation with a plan to have her perform an organic acid test and start a 10-day 4R gut repair program while we waited for the test results.

Two weeks later, we spoke again, and she said she felt a little less depressed, her digestion was improving, and her sinuses were clearing. Reviewing the organic acid test together, I showed her that our assumptions were spot on and that she was showing very low serotonin in her urine. Sharon was pleased and expressed her excitement that finally she had evidence for why her depression was so persistent. I explained to her that a lack of serotonin cannot be fixed by drugs, because they don't treat the cause of the problem. A better idea was to replace the vitamins, amino acids, and cofactors her body needed to make serotonin all by itself. The body wasn't broken; it was just depleted. Sharon agreed and started a targeted protocol to increase tryptophan, 5-HTP, and support MTHFR pathways with B9, B12, and B6.

We gave her four weeks to work with the serotonin support and then reconnected with her. Sharon's face was beaming as she proudly shared with us that for the first time in over a decade she no longer needed to take her medication. She felt better than she had felt in years, with her energy back and a renewed sense of focus and positive energy about life. Last time we spoke, Sharon concluded that she felt so good on the vitamins and supplements that she is planning on staying on them for the foreseeable future. I told her that makes perfect sense, and that by supporting her methylation cycle and providing the serotonin precursors, her depression would be a thing of the past.

One of the best things about studying methylation and epigenetics is that it can accurately explain why things happen. Methylation helps to explain not just why cancer and heart disease are common among certain families, but also why depression is a common finding as well. Sharon's depression wasn't due to the lack of an SSRI; her problem was that she needed her methylation cycle turned on. The issue with depression and MTHFR comes down to the fact that people with slow methylation cannot produce serotonin (and dopamine) as quickly as they need to. But as with Sharon's case, once we optimize the methylation cycle properly, depression often melts away naturally.

The magic of MTFHR and methylation has everything to do with amino acid biochemistry and the production of cofactors. If you remember from biochemistry class, cofactors are ingredients that are required for certain chemical reactions to take place. We couldn't build a wooden house without screws or nails, because these are the cofactors necessary to hold the wood structure in place. It is the same with our own brain's biochemistry. We cannot produce neurotransmitters that speed up our brain and cure depression without amino acids and cofactors from the methylation cycle. Understanding how all these different systems—blood sugar, insulin, amino acids, methylation, and cofactors—come together will be our focus for the next two chapters.

THE HYPOGLYCEMIA PROBLEM

I meet patients every day who have a good diet, but they are not getting better. Despite their healthy diet and avoidance of many foods, they are unable to sleep better, lose weight, increase their energy, and simply feel good. This often happens because their digestive systems and their brains are being shut down by blood sugar problems. Timing our meals correctly and not skipping meals are massively important for the healing process. And let me tell you, skipping meals is a major, major problem in our society!

Sure, high blood sugar and diabetes is a well-known problem and it gets all kinds of attention. The difference between people with high versus low blood sugar is in how quickly they feel symptoms. It may take years to determine that you have high blood sugar, yet every single time your blood sugar drops, you will feel it in a major way. Because of how aggressively the body responds to hypoglycemia, I am convinced that low blood sugar is a worse problem to live with, especially for people with COMT, MAO, and ACE-related genes. In fact, if blood sugar drops too far or too fast, it may even become a life threatening condition.

When I say low blood sugar or hypoglycemia, I don't always mean blood sugar levels below 60 mg/dl. For many people with insulin resistance, blood sugar levels may be ranging from 110 to 180 mg/dl, or higher, throughout the day versus the 70 to 110 mg/dl or so for healthy individuals. When blood sugar levels are averaging 140 mg/dl or more, you don't have to drop the levels all the way down to 65 or 58 mg/dl before you feel symptoms and get a negative reaction. It is the *relative* level of blood sugar that is important. Also, the speed with which the blood sugar levels drop is a huge factor in how it affects your body. If your blood sugar is 140 mg/dl and it drops to 85 mg/dl in just a few minutes, that will create problems just like having your fasting sugars drop into the 50s. In other words, the faster the drop in your sugars, the greater the stress on your body! Figure 9.1 illustrates this concept.

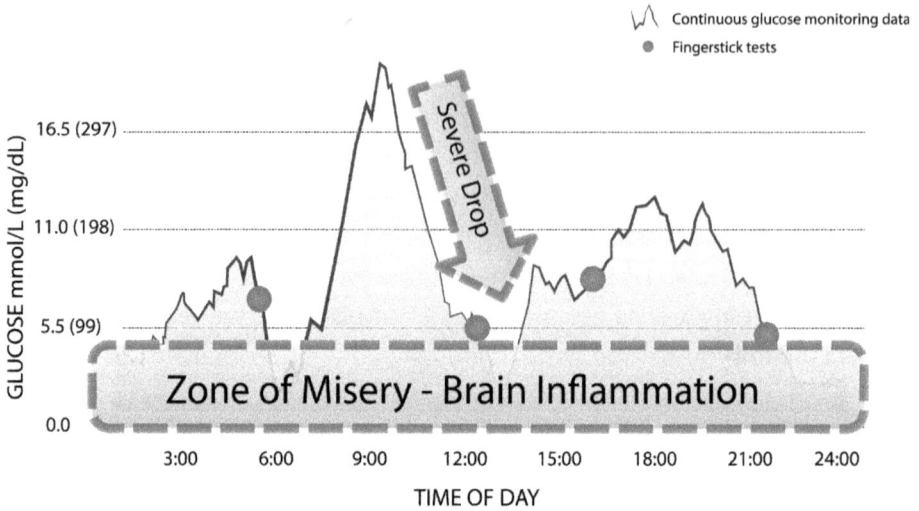

Figure 9.1 - *Overview of how rapid drops in blood sugar damage the body and create brain inflammation. Traditional blood sugar testing often misses the large glucose swings.*

Skipping meals, especially in people with chronic health problems, will trigger a low blood sugar stress reaction, which is often called reactive hypoglycemia. When blood sugar levels drop too fast, an alarm goes off inside our body and we enter what is known as the "zone of misery." To tell the brain that glucose levels are dropping too quickly, a sensor is activated inside the carotid body of the carotid artery.[2] This biochemical sensor is very close to the brain, which helps keep the brain informed of the sugar levels in the blood. This carotid body sensor also requires acetylcholine to function, so individuals who have poor acetylcholine levels will likely also have trouble balancing their blood sugar levels.[3]

Every time we skip a meal, we trigger an adrenal stress reaction from the rapid drop in blood sugar. Our bodies are hard-wired to react to low blood sugar by activating the HPA axis, the Hypothalamic-Pituitary-Adrenal stress system. This fight-or-flight reaction begins with our brain yelling at our adrenal glands and ends with adrenaline and cortisol flooding into our bloodstream. These adrenal hormones are a double-edged sword—they aid us in times of crisis but they can also tear our body apart. And when we chronically skip meals, we do violence to ourselves from the side effects of adrenal stress hormones.

The fact is that adrenaline is very inflammatory, and excess adrenaline will create damaging inflammation in the body. When it breaks down, adrenaline turns into some pretty nasty stuff, like hydrogen peroxide, formaldehyde, and ammonia, which are all toxic to our cells.[4] Studies have proven that adrenaline creates acute inflammation, which can lead to pain, swelling, digestive upset, leaky gut problems, and immune dysfunction.[5, 6] And, again, I have to ask, do we really need more inflammation in our bodies?

TILL PROVEN OTHERWISE

When I first started investigating the phenomenon of low blood sugar, I wanted to find out if there was a common cause to many of the symptoms my patients were experiencing. But it wasn't just my patients who were experiencing these symptoms—I have also struggled with hypoglycemia for years as a child and young adult. Like many people in Western cultures, I grew up on highly processed, high-carbohydrate baby formula. This type of diet creates a hypoglycemia roller coaster pattern of highs and lows, leaving you focused and energetic one minute and then severely fatigued, achy, depressed, and grumpy the next. Though many people might be inclined to blame their COMT, MAO, or MTHFR genes for these symptoms, blood sugar issues are the root cause more than 90 percent of the time.

Reactive hypoglycemia is common for people of all ages, but especially for young children and adolescents who have a much higher metabolism and need for frequent calories. Blood sugar problems are the number one cause of depression and low tryptophan in the brain, a fact that will become apparent as we move through this chapter. You will see how simple processes like insulin and blood sugar have powerful, far-reaching impacts on our brain and digestion, and on every cell and process in our body.

The question naturally arises as to who has a low or a high blood sugar issue. My answer is very simple: Everyone has a problem with their blood sugar levels *until proven otherwise*. I can say this with confidence, not just from my own clinical experience, but also by looking at the most recent scientific data surrounding diabetes and obesity.

Americans, and the world as a whole, are more overweight and obese than at any time in history. Today more than 74 percent of Americans are overweight or obese.[7] Incredibly, worldwide, it is now more common for an individual to become ill from being overweight than to suffer from the diseases that result from starvation.[8] We are literally being killed by the calories of convenience!

Clearly, curing hunger is an ongoing struggle, but if starvation is replaced with GMO crops and processed foods with little to no nutritional value and high amounts of poison, we still collectively lose. It is shocking to realize we now face a 50 percent lifetime risk of diabetes and that diabetes costs American society more than $240 billion each year.[9, 10] These statistics indicate that a majority of you reading this book are dealing with prediabetic glucose levels every day!

If we follow standard healthcare advice, we will wait until our glucose problems get bad enough to need medication, creating another lifelong drug customer in the process. Yet by understanding this problem, we can put a stop to it and create an optimum state of health and genetic expression. To me, that sounds like a better idea.

We cannot have a society with sky-high rates of diabetes and obesity without major blood sugar issues. You see, the road to diabetes and high blood sugar always passes through hypoglycemia. It isn't that a diabetic went to bed on Monday without diabetes and woke up on Thursday with full-blown type 2 diabetes. No, it is a process of losing control of blood sugar levels that often takes years to manifest fully as diabetes.

During the prediabetes years, individuals' blood sugar may spike into hyperglycemia with diets comprising refined carbohydrates, processed foods, soda, alcohol, and other bad foods. This spike is followed by an equally rapid drop in blood sugar after the pancreas releases a large dose of insulin to try to deal with the high glucose. Blood sugar spikes up and then down, over and over again, for years, before a formal diagnosis.

Because half of the American population will be diabetic and three-fourths of Americans are overweight or obese, blood sugar must be stabilized in every single person. Treating blood sugar issues isn't as glamorous or technical as working on genetic pathways, but it is arguably more important. To aid you in your blood sugar balancing quest, I have included specific diet, lifestyle, and nutritional protocols at the end of the chapter. Let's now take a look at the symptoms of this common problem we all face.

The symptoms that accompany low blood sugar will be familiar to everyone reading this book. Odds are many of you are living with these blood sugar effects every day. As research consistently points out, the most common symptoms of hypoglycemia are headaches, nausea, weakness, dizziness, diarrhea, rapid heartbeat, and profuse sweating.[11] Blood sugar problems are common in people who consistently wake up in the middle of the night, run out of energy each and every afternoon, and depend on coffee and sugar to wake up every morning. Blood sugar issues cause happy, well-mannered children and adults to regress into crabby, grumpy, and angry shadows of their former selves. Once you know what you are looking for, you will find low blood sugar issues all around you.

LOW BLOOD SUGAR RAISES STRESS AND LOWERS STOMACH ACID PROBLEMS

Along with all the nasty side effects of adrenaline, we experience another problem when we suffer through a period of low blood sugar (hypoglycemia). Our body becomes unable to produce stomach acid. Yes, you heard that right: low blood sugar is a major cause of low stomach acid and weak digestion. It may not be widely known that the same hormones we use when our lives are threatened are used when our blood sugar drops. Yet from our body's point of view, low blood sugar is no less a threat than being chased by a grizzly bear or saber-toothed tiger!

To raise blood sugar, the body releases large amounts of adrenaline and glucagon, two powerful hormones that impact the liver by increasing glucose production. This is called the counterregulatory response.[12, 13] The big problem with this system is that glucagon and adrenaline carry some very strong side effects. Most people don't realize their fatigue, brain fog, poor vision, headaches, and binge eating are mostly side effects of the hormones our body uses to raise our blood sugar levels.

As I have shared with you throughout this book, adrenaline and its sister molecules dopamine and norepinephrine can be very toxic to the brain and body. The adrenaline side effects of anxiety, chronic pain, poor sleep, and poor memory can wreak havoc on our daily lives. Yet it's the other low blood sugar hormone, glucagon, that is a main problem for our stomach function.

Many of you may not have heard of glucagon, but it's an easy hormone to understand. Think of glucagon as a hormone that is the opposite of insulin—it literally means glucose "be gone" from the cell. In other words, insulin is used by the body to lower blood sugar levels, and glucagon is used by the body to raise blood sugar levels. Pretty simple. Interestingly, although they have opposite functions in the body, they both come from the same organ—the pancreas.

When our blood sugar drops during periods of fasting, the body doesn't need much insulin, so the pancreas doesn't release very much. However, when we are fasting and indulging in meal-skipping, the pancreas releases large amounts of glucagon. And the problems for our digestive system show up when glucagon levels rise quickly. First understand that low blood sugar, regardless of the cause, will trigger the pancreas to work very hard to increase levels of glucagon in the bloodstream. In fact, the level of glucagon can rapidly rise up to four times the normal amount as our blood sugar levels drop toward 60 mg/dl.[14] All this glucagon is released because the body is starving for glucose, which is needed to fuel the brain and other important body systems. But that still doesn't explain why it hurts our digestion so much.

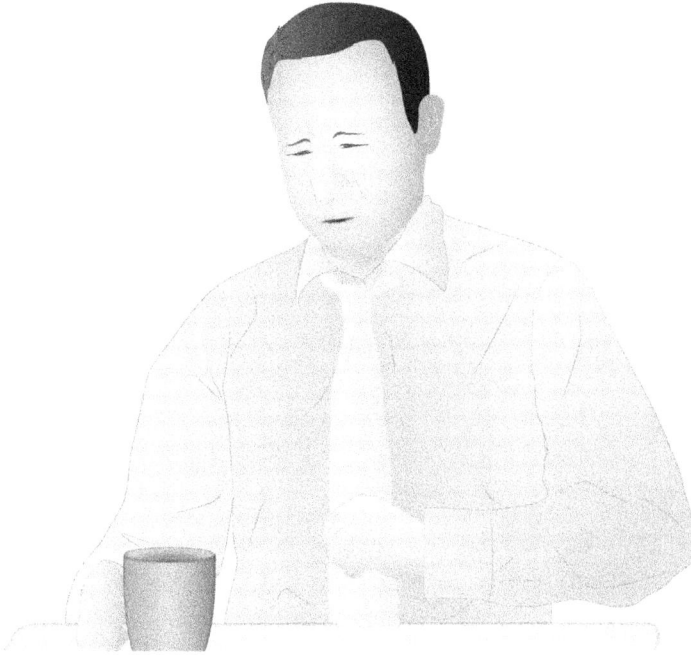

Figure 9.2 - *Hypoglycemia shuts off stomach acid production and leads to poor absorption and common symptoms like acid reflux or GERD.*

The reason that glucagon impairs digestion is that it causes the stomach to stop making stomach acid.[15] Glucagon inhibits the production of hydrochloric acid (HCl), which inhibits digestion, and we know from chapter 4 just how critical digestion is for our optimum health. Although it may not make sense at first, the body always has a reason for doing what it does.

When our blood sugar level is low, our energy is also low. Conserving what little energy is available becomes a priority for the body. Since glucagon is released in high amounts only when blood sugar is low, it carries the message to the stomach to stop making digestive juices because there isn't enough fuel to go around. In this way, glucagon helps to raise blood sugar not just by causing the liver to increase production of glucose, but also by telling a very high energy system like the stomach to shut the factory down until the power comes back online—a genius move by the body, if you ask me.

Even though the body is still acting intelligently by using adrenaline and glucagon, it is possible to experience severe health problems as a result of something as simple as low blood sugar. The relationship between glucose, adrenaline, glucagon, and stomach acid helps to shed light on why hypoglycemia is so bad for our stress levels and our digestive systems. Basically, each and every time we allow our blood sugar to drop (by skipping meals, skipping breakfast, eating a processed-food diet, and other bad habits), we force the pancreas to work overtime, we shut down digestion in the stomach, and we create all kinds of adrenaline-related side effects. So the next time you decide it's a good idea to skip breakfast and then convince yourself you are too busy to stop and eat until dinner, you will understand why this behavior is so health negative!

Now I realize that events such as divorce, illness, job changes, new babies, and others, are very stressful life events. But they don't happen every day. They create massive stress in our lives, but luckily these events are usually few and far between. The same is NOT true for a blood sugar problem. Given the fact that adrenaline and glucagon are released in high amounts, blood sugar stress (low blood sugar) is very likely one of the most stressful things that will ever happen to a person over their lifetime.

Every single day since the moment we were conceived, our blood sugar rises and falls. If we fail to balance our blood sugar through proper food selection and eating frequently, we create an enormous amount of adrenal stress every day! People who don't eat enough or frequently are truly world-class adrenaline junkies. And this can have disastrous consequences on our health, and on the health of those we love.

Sam was a 4-year-old who had struggled with constipation and mood problems most of his life. When his mother spoke with me on the phone, she said that he got very irritable at times throughout the day and he had trouble sleeping. Also, his bowel habits had been very sluggish since he was 2 years old. Some days, he had no bowel movement at all. Other times, he had to sit on the toilet several times a day, sometimes for 30 minutes, before a bowel movement. You don't have to be a doctor to know that is abnormal, especially for a 4-year-old.

Sam's mom also tested his genes with 23andMe.com and gave me a copy of his SNP report she ran through MTHFRSupport.com. He was homozygous (+/+) for COMT and (+) for MAO, and had several other methylation-related markers. I recognized the mood swings were caused by low blood sugar, creating low dopamine in his frontal lobe. His digestive issues were being aggravated by this as well, since a brain without fuel will do a poor job of regulating the gut. Sam wasn't eating frequently enough and he wasn't digesting the food very well. This was making him constipated and ruining his attitude. And this needed to change.

To help prevent his drop in blood sugar throughout the day, I instructed his mom to make sure he ate every 1 ½ to 2 hours, and that he avoided sugars, grains, and sweets that tend to cause reactive hypoglycemia. I also suggested that Sam take a protocol of supplements to help his digestive system and regulate his bowel—things like magnesium-citrate, vitamin C, betaine HCl, probiotics, vitamin D3, and others. I suggested that Sam follow this program for two weeks to determine how we would respond.

At our follow-up phone consultation, Sam's mom was very excited. She related to me how the protocol "hit the nail on the head" and that Sam improved right away. Sam no longer struggled to have a bowel movement and his constipation was a thing of the past. He no longer had to sit on the toilet several times a day. The supplements were well tolerated and he was snacking throughout the day to prevent hunger.

And the best part was that his mood was much better in just a couple weeks. Sam didn't have the usual meltdowns and tantrums he used to have. Instead, he was focused, playful, and a good listener—all signs that his dopamine levels and adrenaline levels were being properly managed.

The key to this case is to see that Sam optimized his genes—the COMT and MAO pathways—by treating his hypoglycemia. This in turn caused his body to produce more dopamine and serotonin at a steady rate throughout the day. Mom was happy because her little angel was acting like one. Sam was happy because he didn't have to spend hours on the toilet. And it only took two weeks!

When we talk about COMT and MAO genes in the brain (which we discuss in more detail in the final two chapters), what we are really trying to understand is whether the person has high or low dopamine and catecholamines. The SNPs I look at in the COMT and MAO pathways are proven to slow the removal of dopamine and norepinephrine from the frontal lobe of the brain. This means people with COMT and MAO SNPs are accustomed to having higher dopamine and noradrenaline in their brain. Just like anything in life, when you get accustomed to having a high amount of something, it really hurts when your levels drop.

The problem with hypoglycemia is that it dramatically lowers the dopamine levels in the brain. People with COMT and MAO genes are genetically inclined to have higher dopamine levels in the frontal lobe, all things being equal. Since they are programmed to work with higher levels of dopamine, they are not equipped to handle a dopamine famine. The brain's dopamine levels drop when blood sugar drops. And the reason why is simple: insulin is required to make dopamine in the brain! (Ding! Ding! Ding!)

THE INSULIN/BLOOD SUGAR AND DOPAMINE CONNECTION

Tyrosine, phenylalanine, and tryptophan, the amino acids we covered back in chapter 7, cannot pass the blood brain barrier (BBB). To get into the brain, they must be transported across on what is called the large neutral amino acid (LNAA) transporter. But as with a ferry boat crossing the river, only a certain amount of space is available and there is competition for those parking spots!

When insulin is elevated after a meal, it makes us feel high because dopamine and serotonin levels rise. This is because insulin helps tyrosine, phenylalanine, and tryptophan find a parking spot on the LNAA ferry boat and cross the BBB river. Insulin does this by causing other amino acids to leave the bloodstream, which opens up room on the LNAA transporter. Insulin not only lowers blood sugar by pushing glucose inside our cells, but it also pushes branched-chain amino acids (BCAAs) into the cells.[16, 17, 18, 19, 20] In this way, insulin helps make it more likely that the precursors to dopamine and serotonin get into the brain.

When insulin is low, we get the opposite problem. There is no space on the LNAA ferry for tyrosine, phenylalanine, or tryptophan, so the brain doesn't get what it needs to make dopamine or serotonin. Low insulin essentially starves the brain of dopamine and serotonin. This makes the brain slow down and is probably the number one cause of brain fog. Without dopamine or serotonin, you aren't going to feel smart or sharp, and your memory will fail. Everyone suffers when dopamine is low, but individuals with COMT and MAO genes will see the most negative change from low dopamine.

All this low dopamine and serotonin will cause cravings for food and/or drugs such as sugar and alcohol. It is widely supported that most common drugs, such as marijuana, cocaine, nicotine, morphine, heroin, and methamphetamines, work by raising dopamine.[21, 22, 23, 24, 25] People who are addicted to these substances are simply trying to self-medicate dopamine deficiencies. And when you see people binging on cookies, cake, dessert, chocolate, wine, and the like, you are again seeing someone reacting to low dopamine.[26] The body is craving the fastest method of raising insulin and raising dopamine—and junk food works just as well as drugs!

CONCLUSION

I know this subject well, because for 20 years of my life, I was one of those people fighting with chronic depression (this is a big reason why I became a doctor and dedicated my life to educating people about methylation and the root causes of problems). Our genes alone cannot explain why so many people are now living with chronic depression. Despite the fact that MTHFR and methylation issues increases our risk of depression, most people still experience depression because of untreated blood sugar issues.

Keeping dopamine, adrenaline, and glucagon levels in a normal range requires prudent dietary habits. If we skip meals, our dopamine drops, cravings go up, anger goes up, and stomach function goes down. To keep us alive, our body secretes high amounts of adrenaline and glucagon as our blood sugar drops. This excess adrenaline helps raise blood sugar rapidly, giving the brain what it needs to maintain homeostasis. The glucagon does basically the same thing but also shuts off digestion in the process. Although these chemicals are helpful in raising blood sugar, there are negative side effects of these powerful, mind-altering, and digestion-destroying chemicals.

High dopamine and adrenaline levels from low blood sugar will make your life difficult at best and miserable at worst. You'll experience shakiness, anxiousness, inability to focus, rapid heartbeat, sweating, poor digestion, and more as main side effects of low blood sugar. I cannot emphasize enough that before you start treating the genes, you must make sure you are treating the person. If you get one idea from reading this book, that should be it! And treating the person means making sure that the person eats the right food, that their food is digested properly, and that their meals are frequent through the day. Skipping meals should be avoided at all costs in our modern, high-stress society. Supplements can never fix a bad diet and bad habits, no matter how much we may try.

BLOOD SUGAR, METHYLATION, DEPRESSION PROTOCOL

The protocol to fix the issues discussed in this chapter requires improved dietary habits as well as the use of supplements to support healthy blood sugar and digestion. Because stomach function is greatly hindered by low blood sugar, make sure to address your low stomach acid by following the protocol from chapter 4. Everyone with symptoms of low blood sugar has a problem with low stomach acid until proven otherwise. Also, before you embark on the protocols from this chapter onward, make sure your gut dysfunction (SIBO, oxalates, yeast, etc.) has been addressed. These protocols use methylated B vitamins, and you need to be sure the gut is functional before you use these tools. Otherwise, you'll feed the bad bugs or won't absorb the vitamins. Therefore, I am going to assume you have done your work from the earlier chapters and are ready for what comes next. If not, go back and make sure!

RECOMMENDED LAB TESTING:

I recommend the Routine Blood Tests and the Organic Acid Test in appendix B for assessing the root causes of blood sugar, methylation, and depression issues. To make full use of the information in this book, I recommend following the instructions found in appendix A to get your own detailed genetic report.

NOTE: Some patients are suffering with chronic viral infections that have gone undetected. The symptoms of chronic viral infection can mimic many of the symptoms I discuss in this book. If you have worked with functional medicine doctors, used supplements, and changed your diet but saw little-to-no results, then you may have some kind of chronic viral issue. In appendix B you will find a list of blood tests to discover if you have an undetected viral problem. In that same area, I provide some general information on viral infections, how the methylation cycle influences this process, and which supplements I have found to be the best at helping you get rid of chronic viruses.

HYPOGLYCEMIA DIET ADVICE:

Without a doubt, the biggest influence in our adrenal system and our energy system is blood sugar. Our cells need sugar to produce fuel, and blood sugar swings, especially hypoglycemia, create a feast-and-famine scenario, where the body doesn't work optimally. By the time we feel hunger, we have triggered an avalanche of hormonal changes that releases stress hormones from the adrenal gland. Because hunger is in fact a type of stress, I teach all my patients with hypoglycemic and depression symptoms to eat more often than just three meals per day.

The easiest thing to do to correct low blood sugar is simply to eat more frequently throughout the day to ensure that your body doesn't become stressed between meals. You can do this by rearranging your eating and snacking schedule. Our recommendation to patients who experience the nausea, shakiness, dizziness, moodiness, and general bad-feeling-ness of low blood sugar is to eat at least 100 calories every 90 minutes to 2 hours. This isn't for the rest of your life, but in the early stages of the healing process, eating this frequently is essential.

Avoiding hunger actually allows your adrenal glands to rest and gain strength, further improving your overall health. This means you must eat at least every 2 hours—always snacking on low-glycemic food options and making sure NEVER to let yourself feel hunger. The only time of the day it is appropriate to be hungry is when we are waking up from sleeping (after 12 hours of fasting). The rest of our day should include time for eating and snacking throughout. Just know that when you leave your house for the day, you should always carry some food and water. This way you are never caught unprepared.

When your blood sugar drops, your body cannot properly digest your food. If the blood sugar is dropping every day, with periods of dizziness, vision problems, fatigue, and brain changes, then the digestive system is basically shut off each time you eat. Over time, your body CANNOT absorb nutrients very well. This can end up being the root cause of many ailments, since your body will struggle to be healthy if your digestive system is weakened.

Our brain depends on amino acids from our diet in order to manufacture the dopamine and serotonin that makes us feel our best. The most common condition in people of all ages that impacts our brain function is hypoglycemia. When the insulin levels drop from low blood sugar, the body cannot get tyrosine, phenylalanine, and tryptophan into the brain. This is why people (adults and children) with low blood sugar have major issues with mood, sleep, focus, and anger.

For example, inappropriate anger often occurs when the brain loses dopamine. Dopamine is what gives us a feeling of satisfaction, of reward. When dopamine levels drop, we get angry because it feels like we lost something valuable to us—such as losing a game, a fight, an argument, etc. When our blood sugar level is balanced, we receive even amounts of dopamine, serotonin, etc., into the brain and we sleep, feel, move, think, and heal much better! The same is true of serotonin, which responds very well to balanced blood sugar and eating frequently.

NOTE: *A lot of evidence suggests that periodic fasting is a healthy, anti-cancer lifestyle that improves our long-term health. And I agree with this idea. But for patients with hypoglycemia, depression, and methylation issues that haven't been addressed I DO NOT recommend fasting. Fasting can be used after 6 to 12 months of working on fixing the underlying issues, but not sooner. Many people are simply too sick in the beginning of the healing process to be good candidates for fasting.*

BLOOD SUGAR, METHYLATION, AND DEPRESSION PROTOCOL:

Chromium Picolinate – 1 capsule 2 times per day with meals. Provides the essential mineral chromium, which improves insulin function and helps regulate fat, protein, and carbohydrate metabolism.† (Nutridyn)

Omega PureEPA-DHA 720 – 2 softgels 3 times per day with meals. Pure, clean, and concentrated Omega-3 fish oil that supports optimum brain, immune, and cardiovascular health.† (Nutridyn)

B-Complex – 1 capsule with breakfast and 1 cap[sule with lunch. Well-rounded B complex that provides support for the methylation cycle, energy production, and adrenal hormones.† (NurriDyn)

L-Tyrosine – 1 capsule 3 times per day with meals. Tyrosine is the required building block for both thyroid hormone and dopamine/adrenaline production.† (Nutridyn)

Crave-Curb – 2 capsules 3 times per day with meals. provides amino acids, vitamins, and herbs in a synergistic formula to increase serotonin naturally.† (Nutridyn)

UltraBiotic Daily Multi-Strain – 1 capsule 1 time per day. Comprehensive probiotic support that provides healthy strains of bacteria and helps reduce yeast and bad bugs.† (Nutridyn)

D3 10,000 with K2 – 1 softgel per day with a meal. Provides numerous benefits to the health and function of the GI tract; patients with gut problems are chronically low in fat-soluble vitamins such as D3.† (Nutridyn)

REFERENCES

1. Pet Scan of the Brain for Depression. Mayo Clinic website. www.mayoclinic.org/tests-procedures/pet-scan/multimedia/-pet-scan-of-the-brain-for-depression/img-20007400. Accessed April 10, 2017.

2. Zhang, M., J. Buttigieg, C.A. Nurse. Neurotransmitter mechanisms mediating low-glucose signaling in cocultures and fresh tissue slices of rat carotid body. *J Physiol.* (2007) 578(Pt 3): 735-50.

3. Fitzgerald, R.S., M. Shirahata, I. Chang, et al. The impact of hypoxia and low glucose on the release of acetylcholine and ATP from the incubated cat carotid body. Brain research. (2009) May 13 (1270): 39-44.

4. Yu, P.H., C.T. Lai, D.M. Zuo. Formation of formaldehyde from adrenaline in vivo; a potential risk factor for stress-related angiopathy. *Neurochem Res.* (1997) 22(5): 615-20.

5. Karalis, K.P., E. Kontopoulos, L.J. Muglia, J.A. Majzoub. Corticotropin-releasing hormone deficiency unmasks the proinflammatory effect of epinephrine. *Proc Natl Acad Sci USA.* (1999) 96(12): 7093-7.

6. de Punder, K., L. Pruimboom. Stress induces endotoxemia and low-grade inflammation by increasing barrier permeability. *Front Immunol.* (2015) 6: 223.

7. Yang, L., G.A. Colditz. Prevalence of overweight and obesity in the United States, 2007-2012. *JAMA Internal Medicine.* (2015) 175(8): 1412-13.

8. Maffetone, P.B., I. Rivera-Dominguez, P.B. Laursen. Overfat and underfat: new terms and definitions long overdue. *Frontiers in Public Health.* (2017) 4: 279.

9. American Diabetes Association. Economic costs of diabetes in the U.S. in 2012. *Diabetes Care.* (2013) 36(4): 1033-46.

10. Gregg, E.W., Xiaohui Zhuo, Yiling J. Cheng, et al. Trends in lifetime risk and years of life lost due to diabetes in the USA, 1985-2011: a modelling study. *The Lancet Diabetes & Endocrinology,* (2014) 2(11): 867-74.

11. Andrade, H.F., W. Pedrosa, F. Diniz Mde, V.M. Passos. Adverse effects during the oral glucose tolerance test in post-bariatric surgery patients. *Arch Endocrinol Metab.* (2016) 60(4): 307-13.

---

12. Verberne, A.J., W.S. Korim, A. Savetghadam, I.J. Llewellyn-Smith. Adrenaline: insights into its metabolic roles in hypoglycaemia and diabetes. *Br J Pharmacol.* (2016) 173(9): 1425–37.

13. Sprague, J.E., A.M. Arbeláez. Glucose counterregulatory responses to hypoglycemia. *Pediatr Endocrinol Rev.* (2011) 9(1): 463–75. PMCID: PMC3755377

14. Guyton, A.C., J.E. Hall. *Textbook of Medical Physiology*, 11th ed. Philadelphia, PA: Elsevier (2006) p. 971.

15. Ibid., p. 970.

16. Fernstrom, J.D. Large neutral amino acids: dietary effects on brain neurochemistry and function. *Amino Acids.* (2013) 45(3): 419-30.

17. Scarna, A., S.F. McTavish, P.J. Cowen, et al. The effects of a branched chain amino acid mixture supplemented with tryptophan on biochemical indices of neurotransmitter function and decision-making. *Psychopharmacology.* (2005) 179(4): 761–8.

18. McTavish, S.F., M.H. McPherson, C.J. Harmer, et al. Antidopaminergic effects of dietary tyrosine depletion in healthy subjects and patients with manic illness. *The British Journal of Psychiatry.* (2001) 179(4): 356–60.

19. Scarna, A., H.J. Gijsman, S.F. McTavish, et al. Effects of a branched-chain amino acid drink in mania. *The British Journal of Psychiatry.* (2003) 182(3): 210–3.

20. Fernstrom, J.D. Branched-chain amino acids and brain function. *The Journal of Nutrition.* (2005) 135(6): 1539S-46S.

21. Mansvelder, H.D., D.S. McGehee. Long-term potentiation of excitatory inputs to brain reward areas by nicotine. *Neuron.* (2000) 27(2): 349-57.

22. Fitzgerald, P.J. Elevated norepinephrine may be a unifying etiological factor in the abuse of a broad range of substances: alcohol, nicotine, marijuana, heroin, cocaine, and caffeine. *Substance Abuse. Research and Treatment.* (2013) 7: 171–83.

23. Bloomfield, M.A., C.J. Morgan, S. Kapur, et al. The link between dopamine function and apathy in cannabis users: an [18F]-DOPA PET imaging study. *Psychopharmacology.* (2014) 231(11): 2251–9.

24. Zald, D.H., R.L. Cowan, P. Riccardi, et al. Midbrain dopamine receptor availability is inversely associated with novelty-seeking traits in humans. *Journal of Neuroscience.* (2008) 28(53): 14372–8.

25. Park, K., N.D. Volkow, Y. Pan, et al. Chronic cocaine dampens dopamine signaling during cocaine intoxication and unbalances D1 over D2 receptor signaling. *Journal of Neuroscience.* (2013) 33(40): 15827–36.

26. Volkow, N.D., G.J. Wang, R.D. Baler. Reward, dopamine and the control of food intake: implications for obesity. *Trends in Cognitive Sciences.* (2011) 15(1): 37–46.

10.

BEYOND BLOOD SUGAR: UNDERSTANDING THE TRYPTOPHAN STEAL AND BH4

The hardest thing to see is what is in front of your eyes.

—Johann Wolfgang von Goethe

As we begin this chapter about depression and tryptophan, I want to ask a simple, but serious, question: Are we programmed to be depressed? The answer to this question will help to explain why we, our loved ones, and our friends all tend to act the way we do. It can shed light on why many people suffer with mental health issues that never seem to be adequately addressed and the reason why millions of Americans are prescribed antidepressants each year in a seemingly endless battle with feeling down, blue, and unhappy.

The answer, unfortunately, is yes. Though it may be hard to believe that our genius body is programmed for depression, that is what the best science and research clearly show. I don't mean that we are *supposed* to be depressed, that we are *destined* to be depressed: In fact, it's quite the contrary. We are supposed to be happy and balanced, level-headed, and relaxed most of the time—except our modern, stressful, and toxic world makes it very difficult for that to happen without us having to work diligently toward a healthy lifestyle, optimum genetic expression, and spiritual wellness. Not only does our modern environment present new and frightening challenges for our bodies to cope with, but we also must deal with the myriad genetic variations carried in each of us that can influence our body's growth, repair, detoxification, and more. Understanding how genetic variations and environmental influences make us sick is a key factor that enables us to heal and move forward. And this is especially true for anyone seeking to heal the root causes of their depression.

Fact is, low blood sugar, stress, and inflammation can have powerful and widespread effects on our levels of serotonin, melatonin, and dopamine. Every system—from the brain, to the gut, to our hormones—is susceptible to the negative effects of low neurotransmitters. This problem is so common that it is easily missed by both patients and doctors. By applying the information in this chapter, you will no longer be living in the dark ages of guessing about depression. You'll learn about the science and some protocols that offer solutions to make your struggles with depression a thing of the past.

FOLATE AND BH4

We start by turning our attention back to the methylation cycle; you know that methylation is required to produce neurotransmitters such as serotonin and dopamine. Although methylation is a big part of making neurotransmitters, it is only part of the recipe. To make our brain chemicals, we need another key ingredient: the essential biomolecule BH4. BH4 is the cofactor that does the heavy lifting in the brain. When it comes to making dopamine and serotonin, activated folate loads the gun and BH4 pulls the trigger. Figure 10.1 gives you a visual of how methylation impacts neurotransmitters and an overview of how folate and BH4 work together.

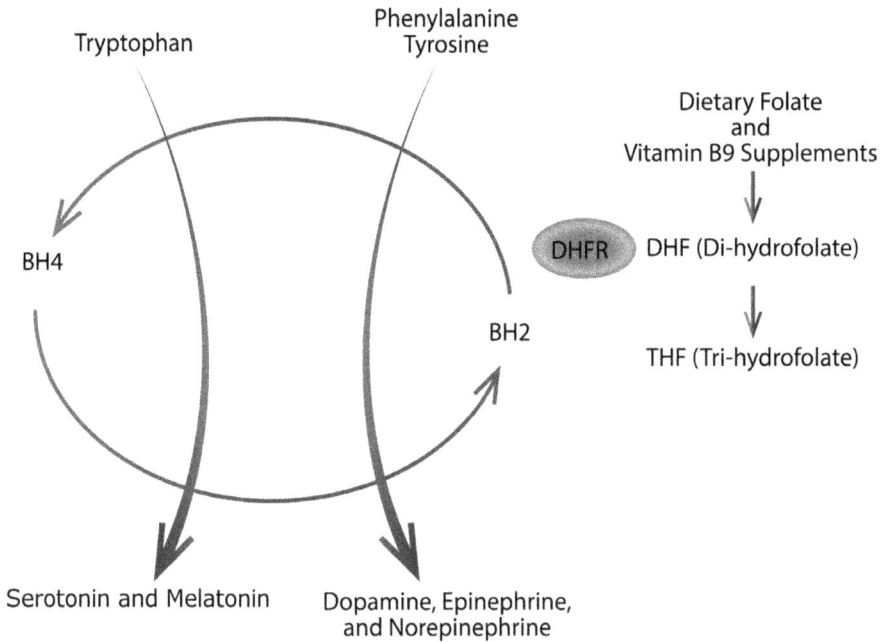

Figure 10.1 – *The BH4 cycle, showing how folate is required to produce neurotransmitters*

The reason why methylation support, especially activated folate (aka 5-MTHF), is so important for depression is because these vitamins increase BH4 levels.[1] Whether the folate comes from our diet or from our gut (remember gut bugs produce folate vitamins) doesn't matter; the fact is that vitamin B9 is required to recycle and increase BH4 levels. Most of the BH4 in our body comes from the methylation cycle, where a folate molecule is used to turn BH2 into BH4.[2, 3] The methylation of BH2 into BH4 provides the cofactor necessary to turn tryptophan and tyrosine into their respective neurotransmitters, serotonin and dopamine. This is how the methylation cycle helps our brain manufacture serotonin and dopamine. Methylation support helps eliminate depression because it enables more BH4 to be produced, which increases neurotransmitters.

The more BH4 we make, the more our brain is able to convert tryptophan into serotonin. And we want that, because more serotonin means less depression, better sleep, and higher libido. This is the real reason why MTHFR genes impact depression so much. People who are born with MTHFR

C677T genes experience a much higher risk of depression. The science is very clear that MTHFR C677T genes are a major risk factor for depression, increasing the risk of depression by a whopping 500 percent![4] But what isn't as well known is that low levels of BH4, resulting from low activated folate, is the real reason why MTHFR problems increase depression. Look again at figure 10.1, and you can see that folate and BH4 team up to help make our happy brain chemicals.

Because BH4 levels are the required cofactors to produce serotonin and dopamine and prevent depression, anything that lowers our BH4 levels will increase our risk of depression. MTHFR genes such as C677T and A1298C are a big problem, because they reduce the amount of folate available and active within our cells. Without a strong MTHFR system in our cells, we cannot activate folic acid and other folate molecules into the form of B9 our body needs—5-MTHF. This leads to a folate deficiency, which can impact all areas of our body, especially our brain. As the body struggles to activate folate through the slowed MTHFR pathways, we produce less BH4 as less vitamin B9 is available in our cells. The bottom line is that without folate, we just don't make much serotonin or dopamine.

Science has known this for some time, but only now are people learning about the power of the methylation cycle to influence the brain. I meet patients every week who are depressed, sleeping poorly, and have low libidos and chronic fatigue. Some of these individuals are aware of the role MTHFR and methylation plays in their condition, while others are not. I explain to each patient that one of the main causes of their depression is a slowed methylation pathway, and that they can bypass the blockage by taking activated nutrients. We know that insulin and blood sugar are key players for healthy brain balance, but so, too, is adequate methylation support for anyone who is dealing with depression.

As many of you know, depression is one of the most misunderstood and poorly treated health conditions in our modern age. Yet depression isn't the monster it appears to be. Like all health problems, depression has a root cause, and once the root cause is addressed, amazing things happen. We just discussed how BH4 and methylation imbalances make us more susceptible to depression, but our genes alone cannot explain why so many people suffer with chronic depression. There is more to depression than bad genes.

You know that genetic problems show up in a big way when we are under stress. Genes react to the environment in either healthy or unhealthy ways, depending on the signals we give them via our thoughts, choices, diet, and lifestyle. When we understand the environment and how it impacts our genetic response, we begin to take control of our destiny. With that in mind, let's focus on tryptophan. There is more to depression than just low blood sugar and a lack of methyl donors and BH4; a lack of tryptophan in the brain can also result in depression! People with depression simply don't have enough tryptophan to go around.[5]

DESTINED TO BE DEPRESSED: THE TRYPTOPHAN STEAL

We humans are not destined to be depressed, but our bodies have developed a sort of biochemical reflex, an automatic response, to toxins, stress, and inflammation that create depression. In other words, *depression results when our body sacrifices our supply of tryptophan as a result of being under stress of any form*. I say *stress in any form* because the research literally shows it doesn't matter whether you are worried about your mortgage, planning a wedding, mourning the loss of a loved one, recovering from food poisoning, sleeping poorly, or dealing with a chronic leaky gut issue. Each one of these problems, and many more, represents a condition in which the body will be forced to sacrifice serotonin in the brain so that cells have a better chance of survival. Under common, everyday conditions of stress, our bodies are programmed to *steal* tryptophan away from the production of serotonin. I call this phenomenon the *Tryptophan Steal*.

There are three common causes of Tryptophan Steal:

- **Adrenal stress**: We live in a very stressful society full of toxins, busy schedules, economic challenges, divorce, and terrorism, to name a few. Each of these factors triggers a powerful, ancient reflex in the brain that causes the adrenal glands to activate. If the adrenal glands are constantly being activated, they enter what is called the *adrenal stress reaction*. This reaction creates wild swings in cortisol levels, which impact all areas of our body, especially our brain, energy, and mood. High cortisol from adrenal stress is a major cause of low serotonin and a big player in the Tryptophan Steal.

- **Blood sugar levels**: You know that blood sugar problems such as diabetes involve high levels of insulin and glucose. And after reading chapter 9, you also know that people with blood sugar issues often experience hypoglycemia or low blood sugar, which actually lowers insulin and glucose, but raises glucagon levels, another powerful hormone from the pancreas. High levels of glucagon can devastate our tryptophan supplies and lead to low serotonin, depression, and poor sleep.

- **Inflammation**: It is no secret that inflammation makes us feel bad. The pain, stiffness, and achiness that accompanies inflammation can put a damper on our mood. Inflammation doesn't just make our body hurt; it also has a huge impact on our brains by changing the chemistry of our nervous systems. An activated, irritated, and inflamed immune system releases hundreds of chemicals, called cytokines, which can trigger the Tryptophan Steal in our brain. The result of all this inflammation isn't just pain, swelling, achiness, and fatigue; it literally changes our brain chemistry and makes us depressed.

These three causes of the Tryptophan Steal are increasingly common. Adrenal stress is being called the "black plague of the 21st century" and is directly responsible for illnesses such as stroke, heart disease, cancer, and even back pain.[6] Diabetes rates continue to climb in the United States, with about 30 million people—about 10 percent of the population of the United States—diagnosed with full-blown diabetes.[7] This number might seem too high, but, sadly, the actual numbers are probably even higher. The *Journal of the American Medical Association* published a report in 2015 showing that approximately 50 percent of all adults in the United States have diabetes or prediabetes.[8] Today, around 150 million people suffer from blood sugar issues, and this health crisis is going to get worse before it gets better. With half the population well on their way to diabetes, and just about everyone fighting off the negative effects of stress, it's no wonder that Big Pharma is making a killing selling us drugs for depression.

While those statistics are a bit disturbing and deserve our attention, we also need to look at the impact of inflammation. Most of us have felt a sore throat from a cold virus or the swelling and itching of a bug bite. These symptoms of inflammation are not caused by a bug or virus per se; they are caused by the body's autoimmune response to the toxic insult. As with stress and blood sugar problems, the rates of autoimmune diseases (in which the body's immune system attacks healthy tissues) are skyrocketing. Recent estimates suggest that 24 to 50 million Americans currently live with some form of an autoimmune condition.[9, 10] That means one of out every six Americans is walking around with some kind of inflammatory immune system disorder.

With millions and millions of people living with chronic problems of stress, blood sugar, and inflammation that can destroy tryptophan levels, it is no wonder depression is so common. Luckily, however, it's not all doom and gloom, because simple, natural solutions can reverse depression naturally by treating the cause—the Tryptophan Steal. And my advice for treating the Tryptophan Steal can be found in the protocols section at the end of this chapter.

AN OVERVIEW OF THE TRYPTOPHAN STEAL

With Tryptophan Steal, the body steals tryptophan from one pathway to give to another. But it isn't a theft of malice; it's an expression of the body's wisdom, of its genius, in managing the limited resource of tryptophan. The body is doing an excellent job of putting its limited supply of tryptophan to use where it is most needed. Figure 10.2 shows the idea more clearly.

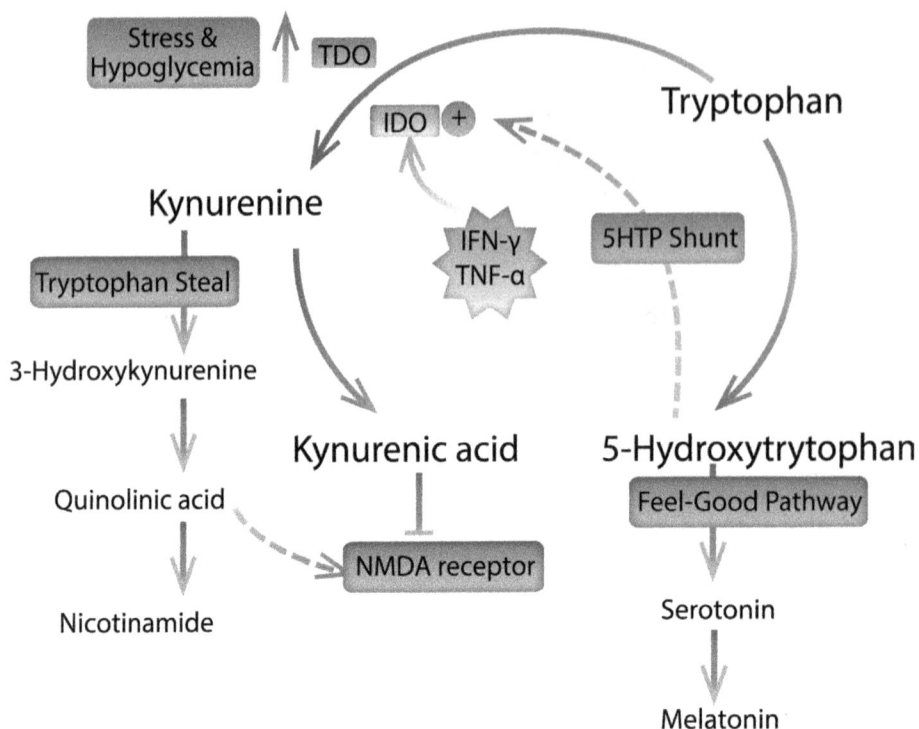

Figure 10.2 – *An overview of the Tryptophan Steal shows how the IDO and TDO enzymes are able to steal tryptophan and 5-HTP and push it down the pathway to make vitamin B3.*

As you can see in the figure, tryptophan follows two main pathways inside the body. On one hand, tryptophan can be turned into 5-HTP, an amino acid that creates serotonin and then turns into melatonin. This is the pathway that helps us make the neurotransmitters that improve our sleep, our energy, and our libido—what I call the "feel-good pathway." On the other hand, tryptophan gets pushed into the pathway that is used to produce vitamin B3, CO^2, and ATP. This second pathway is the kynurenine (ky-nur-e-neen) pathway, and it is the crime scene where the Tryptophan Steal takes place. This kynurenine pathway normally consumes about 95 percent of all the tryptophan in our bodies, with only 1 or 2 percent of tryptophan being used to produce serotonin and melatonin.[11] This second pathway holds our tryptophan hostage and creates problems for those of us suffering with depression. When tryptophan is stolen away from the feel-good pathway, we feel bad—irritated, depressed, anxious, and generally not our best.

Fortunately, you don't have to be a biochemical scientist to understand how this works. The body steals tryptophan from our brain in a straightforward way: The enzymes TDO and IDO, shown in Figure 10.2, are responsible for the Tryptophan Steal. These two enzymes normally help to make sure our cells get enough tryptophan so they can grow, repair, and reach optimum function. However, if stress, inflammation, or blood sugar problems enter the picture, the volume on these two enzymes gets turned way up and our serotonin and melatonin levels get pushed way down. In other words, the body uses these two enzymes to steal tryptophan when necessary. They push tryptophan into the kynurenine pathway to make more NAD and ATP at the expense of our calming, feel-good neurotransmitters.

These two enzymes are very sensitive to changes in their environment, and the greater the biochemical stress, the faster these enzymes will go. Published biochemical research helps us see this idea more clearly. In a study published in 2014, researchers highlighted how the TDO enzyme is activated by cortisol (stress) and low blood sugar swings (glucagon), while the IDO enzyme is turned on by inflammation.[12] Thus cortisol, glucagon, and inflammation can each flush tryptophan levels down the drain and destroy our serotonin levels; and when this happens we often lose our sense of well-being.

NAD AND VITAMIN B3

So now you understand that stress, hypoglycemia, and inflammation cause the Tryptophan Steal, and that causes depression. I could probably stop here and call it good, but there is a key part of this story I have yet to discuss: how demand for the vitamin called *nicotinamide adenine dinucleotide* (NAD) causes the body to steal your tryptophan in the first place. You may remember we briefly touched on NAD back in chapter 7. Recall that NAD is a fascinating chemical that is made from vitamin B3. Since tryptophan is the only method used by the body to make B3, we know that tryptophan is very, very important for NAD production. And you will soon see why NAD levels are a big deal for our health, our brain, and our cells.

NAD is a catalyst in the mini-nuclear reactors in our cells—the mitochon-

dria. NAD plays a role in the movement of electrons inside the mitochondria, which is essential for
the cell to produce
energy. Normally, our cells
produce plenty of energy
when oxygen and vitamins are
abundant. During times of low
stress, low inflammation, and
optimum blood sugar bal-
ance, our cells receive all the
oxygen and nutrients they
need to create an abundance
of energy. High levels of NAD
are not needed during the
easy times, because the cells'
mitochondria can harvest an
enormous amount of energy
from burning oxygen for fuel.

Why the Body Steals Tryptophan

*Because the body cannot make tryptophan,
when there isn't enough to share, the body
steals tryptophan from neurotransmitter
pathways to make more NAD.*

*Stress, blood sugar swings, and inflammation
lower oxygen inside cells, increasing the need
for NAD, which comes only from tryptophan.*

*The tryptophan supply is essential. Ultimately,
the body would rather its cells increase
NAD levels and survive, instead of making
serotonin, sleeping well, and enjoying a good
libido while cells are being destroyed.*

However, as soon as glucagon, cortisol, or inflammation levels increase, the cells begin to lose oxygen and nutrients. Under conditions of stress with low oxygen and low nutrition, cells must use NAD to continue to produce energy, or else they will perish.[13] NAD has a unique capacity to allow our cells' mitochondria to continue to produce energy in the absence of oxygen. This is a handy trait given that *energy is life*, and the more energy our cells make, the better we feel. Whenever the body becomes low in NAD, it will turn on the Tryptophan Steal as a means to survive. So the body has a good reason for stealing your tryptophan—it just doesn't feel very good while it's happening!

Remember that the body doesn't make mistakes—it is too genius for that. It has a very good reason for stealing tryptophan away from serotonin and using it to make NAD. When the body is stressed with adrenal hormones, inflammation, and low blood sugar, cell oxygen levels drop. Without oxygen, cells cannot produce energy very efficiently and will die. To prevent the destruction of our cells when oxygen is low, our body uses NAD to produce energy even during times of stress and low oxygen. Because NAD and serotonin both come from tryptophan, the body has to choose where its bank account of tryptophan will be spent. Lucky for us, the body always chooses right.

Energy is life. And NAD levels will ultimately determine whether our cells survive or perish. In fact, NAD isn't just a vitamin; it also helps our cells acting as an antioxidant, improving cell survival and even preventing auto-immunity.[14, 15, 16] NAD is so powerful that new research is looking at NAD as the proverbial "fountain of youth" and anti-aging molecule.

Researchers have discovered that injecting NAD into 22-month-old mice changes their muscle tissue back to that of a mouse just 6 months old.[17, 18] It's pretty amazing that NAD, which comes from tryptophan, seems to reverse the aging process. It's also interesting that depression makes you feel old and tired. Maybe we should look at giving people with depression support for their NAD levels instead of drugs to mask the symptom. What do you think?

EPIGENETICS AND DEPRESSION GENES: MAO-A AND MAO-B

How can someone have low serotonin if they are homozygous (+ for men or +/+ for women) on their MAO gene? In other words, how can people with a slowed version of MAO rs6323 (the most influential SNP) end up with low serotonin? Doesn't having an MAO SNP mean you are going to have more serotonin, not less? These are all great questions that I hear often, and I asked them myself years ago as I began to study this subject in earnest.

What is missing from these questions is an understanding of something I have repeated throughout my Beyond MTHFR blog and mentioned many times in this book. Our genes are not static, and the environment is always changing how our genes express. You may be born with a certain SNP that predicts something should happen more often, such as low serotonin, but the environment ultimately rules the roost. Nurture beats nature 95 percent of the time.

I have seen this concept in action in my own life and in the lives of thousands of patients I have been fortunate enough to meet. To clarify this idea, let's look at a couple of powerful research studies. One critical study in 2004 blew my mind when I read it. Researchers used a model of inflammation from our immune system and measured how it impacted the genetic expression of the MAO enzyme. These researchers exposed human cells to the Th2 cytokines (immune system chemicals) called IL4 and IL6 and noticed that MAO-A expression was increased more than 2000-fold, or 200,000 percent, while MAO-B showed no noticeable increase.[19]

This proves, in an elegantly simple fashion, that the environment is in control of our genes, especially for key genes related to depression. Interestingly, MAO-A and the cytokines they studied, IL4 and IL6, are associated closely with histamine problems. People with histamine intolerance and chronic histamine symptoms (that is, people with allergies) are known to have an excess of the Th2 cytokines IL4 and IL6.[20, 21] So not only do we have a study giving us clear evidence of the process of epigenetics, but we have a better understanding of why people with histamine issues are also depressed, with low tryptophan. But that isn't all this study shows.

Another takeaway from this study is to recognize that MAO-A was massively upregulated by these inflammatory signals, while MAO-B wasn't affected at all. I realize many of you aren't epigenetic science nerds like me, and you don't speak the scientific language as part of your everyday life. So let me clarify what I mean by MAO-A and MAO-B.

These two genes are very similar but have slightly different shapes, which is why scientists gave them different names. They also have different preferences for neurotransmitters. For example, MAO-A is really, really hungry for serotonin, while MAO-B isn't especially interested in breaking down serotonin. MAO-B prefers dopamine and other lesser known neurotransmitters that are outside of our discussion.

In fact, MAO-A is so hungry for serotonin, that, according to studies, MAO-A has 120 times more affinity for serotonin than MAO-B.[22] So if MAO-A already has a 12,000 percent greater hunger for serotonin, we can only imagine what happens when inflammation increases the expression of MAO-A by an additional several orders of magnitude. You don't have to be a PhD scientist to determine what will follow.

When MAO-A is upregulated (increased) by inflammation, it will literally devour any and all serotonin in the vicinity. It will trigger the mother of all Tryptophan Steals. This is why those who are dealing with excess inflammation are simultaneously dealing with low serotonin and chronic depression. This is why we cannot fix depression without treating the underlying inflammation!

FINDING THE TRYPTOPHAN STEAL ON THE ORGANIC ACID TEST

I am a big fan of the Organic Acid Test from Great Plains Laboratory, and this is especially true as I treat cases of depression. Though I discuss this test in the appendix, I'll cover it briefly here as a means to measure depression.

The Organic Acid Test reveals the evidence of the Tryptophan Steal. After looking at hundreds of these tests, I began to see what the body was trying to do with our neurotransmitters. I knew all the data on tryptophan, MAO enzymes, and depression was important, but until I started seeing the same pattern repeat on hundreds of these tests, I didn't know I was looking at a powerful, preprogrammed reflex: the Tryptophan Steal.

With so much of our body's tryptophan devoted to the kynurenine pathway (95 percent) and so little devoted to the production of serotonin and melatonin (1–2 percent), it doesn't take much to disrupt our brain's level of feel-good neurotransmitters. Imagine if the body needed more NAD and had to shift, or steal, more tryptophan than normal. That might lower available tryptophan from 1.0 to 0.1 percent, or even lower. With only 0.1 percent of tryptophan available for serotonin, it would be like living on only 10 percent of your usual income—that wouldn't be good for your budget or your brain!

The Tryptophan Steal undoubtedly is one of the main causes of chronic insomnia, chronic fatigue, and even chronic pain that I often see in my patients. Each year, I see hundreds of Organic Acid Test results from my patients, and I find that more than 75 percent of them have evidence of the Tryptophan Steal. It is not exactly a "rare" problem. Many patients have serotonin levels in their urine that are very, very close to or actually zero. Not only that, they also often have high levels of quinolinic acid, which is the neurotoxin that can build up if the body's NAD levels are too low and the Tryptophan Steal is activated in earnest.[23] As you can see in Figure 10.3, the Tryptophan Steal is easy to see once you know what to look for.

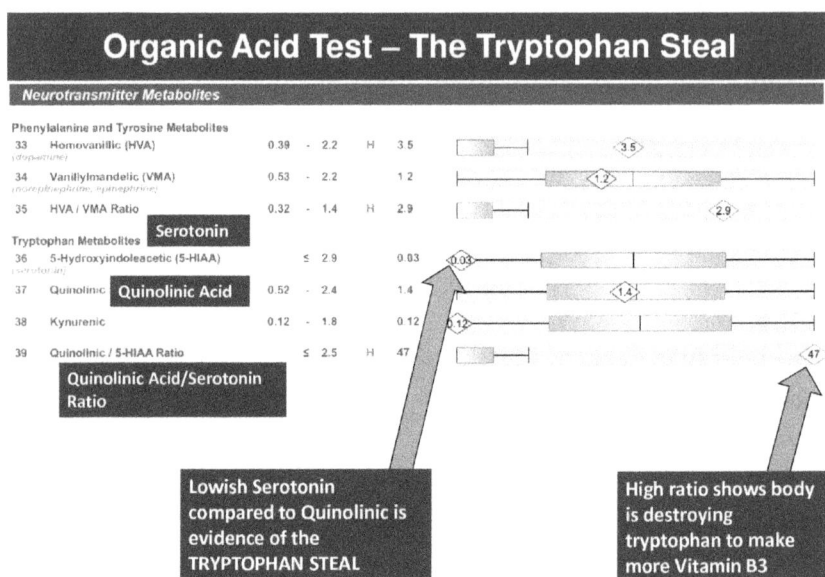

Figure 10.3 - *Great Plains Laboratory Organic Acid Test showing the biochemical evidence of the Tryptophan Steal*

At first blush, you might question why the body would create depression automatically in response to stress, but looking deeper, you can see the genius of the body's design. Given that NAD is needed to keep our cells alive, the body is acting intelligently. The body basically decides that sleeping well, having a healthy sex drive, and being mentally relaxed is not as important as preventing cell destruction. When forced to choose between survival or comfort, the body always makes the right choice.

Thus, we can see that the Tryptophan Steal is a smart adaptation to common stressors. Those of us who have battled depression know the pain and anguish it causes, but those problems are still mild compared to living in a body without adequate levels of NAD. The body is still making the *intelligent* choice, even though it sours our mood and outlook on life. That is still less of a health problem than developing a mitochondrial disorder or suffering from the diarrhea, dermatitis, dementia, and even death, that comes from vitamin B3 deficiency!

CONCLUSION

In this in-depth look at the root cause of depression, the Tryptophan Steal, we discussed how folate increases our BH4 levels so we can turn the amino acids tyrosine and tryptophan into neurotransmitters. We looked at how modern life creates a perfect storm of stress, blood sugar problems, and inflammation that drastically impact our brain and neurotransmitter pathways. If we can agree that every single person on Earth has experienced at least one of these health challenges, we are also agreeing that everyone is potentially at risk for suffering depression.

How long do we experience stress in our lives? Is it for hours, days, months, or years? If the Tryptophan Steal happens for only a short time and you have a balanced methylation cycle with a healthy gut, there is only a small chance that depression will become part of your life. However, if you are like me, with years of chronic stress, poor diet, and gut inflammation, it's almost a guarantee that your body's tryptophan is being stolen and your serotonin levels are low. Everything happens in our body for a reason, and depression has a cause that we know now is the Tryptophan Steal!

TRYPTOPHAN STEAL AND BH4 PROTOCOL

The way to treat the Tryptophan Steal is to make sure the body gets an adequate supply of vitamin B3. In addition to giving the body a therapeutic dose of B3, we need to limit stress, balance blood sugar, and reduce inflammation, since these are the root causes of the Tryptophan Steal. If you have taken my advice so far in this book, then you have already been treating those root causes pretty well. Also, it bears repeating that the gut repair process from chapters 4–7 is key to effectively treat brain-based issues such as depression, anxiety, and other mood issues. A sick gut cannot provide adequate nutrition to help heal the brain.

RECOMMENDED LAB TESTING:

I recommend the Routine Blood Tests and the Organic Acid Test in appendix B for assessing the Tryptophan Steal and other serotonin-related compounds. To make full use of the information in this book, I recommend following the instructions found in appendix A to get your own detailed genetic report.

TRYPTOPHAN STEAL PROTOCOL:

The goal with these supplements is to provide therapeutic levels, 1000–2000mg per day, of niacinamide to help the body produce more NAD inside the cells. Improving NAD levels allows tryptophan and serotonin levels to rise. Niacinamide is a form of B3 that can be taken in high doses without causing a flush. The following supplements are my two favorite tools for supporting the need for increased B3 levels. Choose one from the list.

NAC-600 Mg – 2 capsules 2 times per day with meals. Provides therapeutic levels of N-Acetyl-Cysteine, a cofactor to improve glutathione production.† (Nutridyn)

And

Niacinamide 500 – 1 to 2 capsules 2 times per day with meals. Provides a concentrated dose of niacinamide to improve NAD levels.† (Nutridyn)

---

†This statement has not been evaluated by the FDA. This product is not intended to diagnose, treat, cure, or prevent any disease. The information provided in this book is intended for your general knowledge only and is not a substitute for professional medical advice or treatment for specific medical conditions. You should not use this information to diagnose or treat a health problem or disease without consulting with a

REFERENCES

1. Alkaitis, M.S., M.J. Crabtree. Recoupling the cardiac nitric oxide synthases: tetrahydrobiopterin synthesis and recycling. *Curr Heart Fail Rep*. (2012) 9(3): 200–10.

2. Moens, A.L., C.J. Vrints, M.J. Claeys, et al. Mechanisms and potential therapeutic targets for folic acid in cardiovascular disease. *American Journal of Physiology-Heart and Circulatory Physiology*. (2008) 63(5): H1971.

3. Luiking, Y.C., G.A. Ten Have, R.R. Wolfe, et al. Arginine de novo and nitric oxide production in disease states. *American Journal of Physiology-Endocrinology and Metabolism*. (2012) 303(10): E1177–89.

4. Słopien, R., K. Jasniewicz, B. Meczekalski, et al. Polymorphic variants of genes encoding MTHFR, MTR, and MTHFD1 and the risk of depression in postmenopausal women in Poland. *Maturitas*. (2008) 61(3): 252–5.

5. Maes, M. The cytokine hypothesis of depression: inflammation, oxidative & nitrosative stress (IO&NS) and leaky gut as new targets for adjunctive treatments in depression. *Neuro Endocrinol Lett*. (2008) 29(3): 287–91.

6. Barrow, B. Stress 'is top cause of workplace sickness' and is so widespread it's dubbed the 'black death of the 21st century'. Daily Mail. www.dailymail.co.uk/health/article-2045309/Stress-Top-cause-workplace-sickness-dubbed-Black-Death-21st-century.html. Published October 5, 2011. Accessed September 10, 2016.

7. American Diabetes Association. Statistics about diabetes. www.diabetes.org/diabetes-basics/statistics/. Accessed September 10, 2016.

8. Menke, A., S. Casagrande, L. Geiss, et al. Prevalence of and Trends in Diabetes Among Adults in the United States, 1988-2012. *JAMA*. (2015) 14(10): 1021–9.

9. American Autoimmune Related Diseases Association Autoimmune Statistics - Autoimmune Disease Fact Sheet. www.aarda.org/autoimmune-information/autoimmune-statistics/. Accessed September 10, 2016.

10. National Institute of Environmental Health Sciences. Autoimmune Diseases. www.niehs.nih.gov/health/materials/autoimmune_diseases_508.pdf. Published November 2012. Accessed September 10, 2016.

11. Keszthelyi, D., F.J. Troost, A.A. Masclee. Understanding the role of tryptophan and serotonin metabolism in gastrointestinal function. *Neurogastroenterol Motil*. (2009) 21(12): 1239–49.

---

12. Campbell, B.M., E. Charych, A.W. Lee, et al. Kynurenines in CNS disease: regulation by inflammatory cytokines. *Front Neurosci.* (2014) 8: 12.

13. Penberthy, W.T., I. Tsunoda. The importance of NAD in multiple sclerosis. *Curr Pharm Des.* (2009) 15(1): 64-99.

14. Ayla, S., I. Seckin, G. Tanriverdi, et al. Doxorubicin induced nephrotoxicity: protective effect of nicotinamide. *Int J Cell Biol.* (2011) 2011: 390238.

15. Kolb, H., V. Burkart. Nicotinamide in type 1 diabetes. Mechanism of action revisited. *Diabetes Care.* (1999) 22 Sup 2: B16-20.

16. Suarez-Pinzon, W.L., J.G. Mabley, R. Power, et al. Poly (ADP-ribose) polymerase inhibition prevents spontaneous and recurrent autoimmune diabetes in NOD mice by inducing apoptosis of islet-infiltrating leukocytes. *Diabetes.* (2003) 52(7): 1683-8.

17. Prolla, T.A., J.M. Denu. NAD+ deficiency in age-related mitochondrial dysfunction. *Cell Metab.* (2014) 19(2): 178-80.

18. Mendelsohn, A.R., J.W. Larrick. Partial reversal of skeletal muscle aging by restoration of normal NAD$^+$ levels. *Rejuvenation Res.* (2014) 17(1): 62-9.

19. Chaitidis, P., E.E. Billett, V.B. O'Donnell, et al. Th2 response of human peripheral monocytes involves isoform-specific induction of monoamine oxidase-A. *J Immunol.* (2004) 173(8): 4821-7.

20. Hardy, H., J. Harris, E. Lyon, et al. Probiotics, Prebiotics and Immunomodulation of Gut Mucosal Defences: Homeostasis and Immunopathology. *Nutrients.* (2013) 5(6): 1869-912. PMCID: PMC3725482

21. Diehl, S., M. Rincón. The two faces of IL-6 on Th1/Th2 differentiation. *Mol Immunol.* (2002) 39(9): 531-6. PMID: 12431386

22. Bortolato, M., J.C. Shih. Behavioral outcomes of monoamine oxidase deficiency: preclinical and clinical evidence. *Int Rev Neurobiol.* (2011) 100: 13-42.

23. Lugo-Huitrón, R., P. Ugalde Muñiz, B. Pineda, et al. Quinolinic acid: an endogenous neurotoxin with multiple targets. *Oxidative medicine and cellular longevity.* (2013).

11.

THE GENETIC ROOTS OF PAIN
AND ANXIETY: COMT AND MAO

All illnesses have some heredity contribution. It's been said that
genetics loads the gun and environment pulls the trigger.

—Francis Collins

Although everyone has felt the negative effects of stress in their lives, not everyone responds to stress in the same way. Although our life experience has a great deal of influence on our perception of stress, certain genes make us more or less sensitive to stress. One big reason why stress affects each of us differently has to do with how well our bodies can detoxify catecholamines, the chemicals of stress. And the methylation cycle has a huge influence on how well we both create and detoxify catecholamines. This chapter will show you how an important gene, the COMT gene, controls how the brain reacts to stress. By showing how the COMT gene influences the level of dopamine and adrenaline, it will become clear how important the COMT pathway is for our mental and emotional health.

Specifically, we'll look at the COMT gene and how it influences brain function. This will give you the background necessary to understand why and how stress can change your brain. Because the COMT system is involved in the metabolism and detoxification of stress hormones, it has a major influence on how we deal with stress. Its sister enzyme, MAO, also plays a role here. Research points out that the COMT and MAO enzymes have a huge impact on dopamine levels inside the brain.[1] Therefore, anything that interferes with the function of these enzymes will make you more sensitive to the effects of stress.

NOTE: *For simplicity's sake, I use the terms catecholamines, dopamine, adrenaline, and norepinephrine interchangeably. These terms all relate to the same hormones and neurotransmitters released by our body when it's under stress. If you want to do more research on your own, you will find that there are differences between these chemicals, but for now I am lumping them all together for ease of teaching and understanding.*

When people experience stress, some rally to the cause and increase their performance, while others seem to melt and fall apart under the same type of pressure. How can people undergoing the same type of stress have such different experiences? The answer lies in understanding how the COMT and MAO system influences the brain.

Figure 11.1 shows the complex pathway involved in detoxifying stress hormones. COMT and MAO enzymes are major players in the removal of stress hormones and neurotransmitters. As you will see in the next chapter, sex hormones also interfere with this pathway, making our brains even more susceptible to catecholamine-related illness.

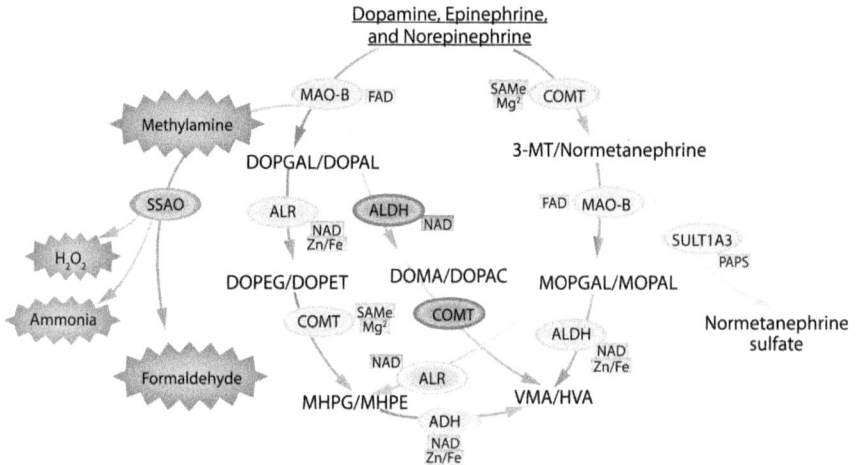

Figure 11.1 – *COMT and MAO Catecholamine Pathway. Ovals represent genes/enzymes and the rectangles adjacent to them list the cofactors necessary to make the enzyme function.*

People with MAO-A and COMT are some of the smartest, most intelligent people you will ever meet. The reason is that these SNPs increase catecholamines in the frontal lobes of our brain. If you are blessed with increased dopamine and adrenaline, you will be able to focus like a laser at times, and you'll usually be very detail oriented with a good memory, as long as the system isn't overstressed. But if your body becomes overstressed from gut inflammation, food allergies, physical exhaustion, too much exercise, vitamin and mineral deficiencies, chronic infections, and the like, you have a recipe for being a stress-mess!

COMT GENE POLYMORPHISMS: A COMMON PROBLEM

The first thing to realize is that COMT gene polymorphisms are very common. I tell my patients with COMT SNPs that they are in good company. This helps to defuse the toxic idea of having a "genetic" problem, and it is not far from the truth. We now know that 80 percent of the European and North American population has a SNP in the COMT V158M gene, which is the COMT gene that has been studied the most. A 2015 study published in Sleep Medicine Reviews highlighted the fact that 30 percent of people in this population are homozygous (+/+) and 50 percent are heterozygous (+/–) for the COMT V158M allele.[2] Amazingly, the same research article also revealed that the COMT V158M polymorphism slows down the COMT system three to four times.[2] If you slow something down in your body four times more than normal, you don't have to be a scientist to know that it can impact your health.

Since the vast majority of people alive today have genetic imbalances in their stress metabolism pathway, we have to ask a few questions:

- If 80 percent of everyone has a COMT gene imbalance, wouldn't you expect that 80 percent of people would have "stress-mess symptoms" such as anxiety, panic, worry, and insomnia, which come from a slowed COMT pathway?

- Wouldn't it make sense that if 80 percent of the population has a slowed COMT pathway, that stress would cause the same symptoms in each person?

- Don't genes control your destiny? For example, if you have alterations in the way your body detoxifies stress hormones, are you not destined to be a "super stress-mess"?

By now, you should know that the answer to each of these questions is a resounding NO!

I love to tell my patients that just because they have a gene for something doesn't mean it will be a problem. In fact, the environment inside the body is many times more important than your genes. Yet we cannot ignore that certain genes do influence how we feel. And without a doubt, the COMT gene has a massive influence on how we feel on a day-to-day basis.

COMT AND THE CATECHOLAMINE BELL CURVE

The COMT system helps to break down dopamine, norepinephrine, and epinephrine, the neurotransmitters our body releases when it is under stress. The brain is a lot like Goldilocks in "The Three Bears" story: it wants just the right amount of stress, not too little, and not too much. In other words, the brain functions on a bell curve of activity, with dysfunction on either end and optimum function in the middle. Figure 11.2 illustrates this point in detail.

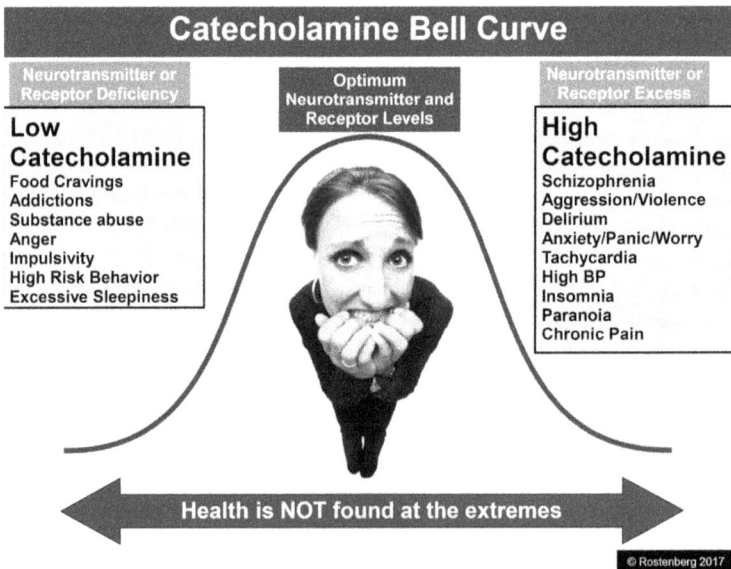

Catecholamine Bell Curve

Neurotransmitter or Receptor Deficiency

Optimum Neurotransmitter and Receptor Levels

Neurotransmitter or Receptor Excess

Low Catecholamine
Food Cravings
Addictions
Substance abuse
Anger
Impulsivity
High Risk Behavior
Excessive Sleepiness

High Catecholamine
Schizophrenia
Aggression/Violence
Delirium
Anxiety/Panic/Worry
Tachycardia
High BP
Insomnia
Paranoia
Chronic Pain

Health is NOT found at the extremes

© Rostenberg 2017

Figure 11.2 – Symptoms of low and high catecholamines

Basically, the "catecholamine bell curve" implies that our dopamine problems in the brain come in two distinct flavors:

- **LOW DOPAMINE or LOW CATECHOLAMINES:** The left side of the bell curve, where dopamine is low, will cause depression of the frontal lobe, slowdown of neuronal circuits, and malfunctions of the neocortex as it slows down too much. Symptoms include the following:

  > Cravings

  > Substance abuse

  > Addictions

  > Anger

  > Impulsivity

  > High risk behavior

  > Poor memory and brain fog

- **HIGH DOPAMINE or HIGH CATECHOLAMINES:** The right side of the bell curve, where there is excess dopamine, causes overstimulation of the frontal lobe, neuronal circuit fatigue from overstimulation, and malfunctions of the neocortex as it fires too fast. Symptoms include the following:*

  > Anxiety

  > Chronic pain

  > Worry

  > Delirium

  > Tachycardia

  > High blood pressure

  > Insomnia

> Paranoia/Mania

> Schizophrenia/Psychosis

> Poor memory and brain fog

It is my clinical opinion that most individuals who experience "overmethylation" symptoms are actually feeling the side effects of excess catecholamines.

When the level of dopamine in the frontal lobe is balanced and optimized, your brain works at its best. In contrast, if dopamine levels in the frontal lobe fall too low, you become depressed, and if they increase too much, you become anxious and worried. Although most symptoms of high catecholamines are different from the symptoms of low catecholamines, you will experience memory loss and brain fog *at both ends of the catecholamine bell curve*. This might seem confusing at first, but remember that whenever the dopamine levels fall too far or rise too high, the brain function declines. When your brain function is compromised, you will have problems with memory (short-term more than long-term) and your thinking and problem-solving processes will feel foggy. These catecholamines are so powerful that when they are out of balance, we are out of balance! It's fair to say that the majority of brain symptoms we face each day result from imbalanced dopamine levels.

Some of you may recognize an apparent contradiction: Some patients experience symptoms from both low and high catecholamine categories. Many patients suffer from both anxiety and depression, and this is a common complaint among my patients. This double complaint has a lot to do with how catecholamine levels change throughout the day. When both serotonin and dopamine are low, we are depressed. When dopamine rises *relative* to serotonin levels, we experience anxiety more than depression. You can wake in the morning depressed, then eat a high sugar diet and abuse caffeine and experience anxiety in the afternoon. This is a very common pattern, and it makes sense when you look at it from the point of view of the catecholamines and serotonin levels.

It is well accepted that low serotonin causes depression, and research supports the idea that dopamine is the main driver of anxiety. Current peer-reviewed studies show us that dopamine is mostly responsible for causing feelings of fear and worry, acting through dopamine receptors in the limbic system to create anxiety.[3, 4] Although I believe more research can help us solve this apparent contradiction, the preceding explanation has made the most sense in explaining how this occurs.

THE ADVANTAGES OF HIGHER DOPAMINE LEVELS

Higher dopamine isn't always a bad thing, however. Remember that when individuals are born with a SNP in the COMT gene (especially the V158M COMT), they are born with a slower COMT enzyme. This predisposes them to having more dopamine in the frontal lobe of the brain. Under less-stressful circumstances, these individuals are proven to have better memory and more brain function—basically, they are very smart people!

Remember, too, that more dopamine in the frontal lobe of the brain offers an advantage in less-stressful periods. With more dopamine (and norepinephrine and epinephrine), individuals have a very alert mind and better memory, and they are quick, sharp learners. With higher dopamine levels, the brain becomes more active, receives more oxygen and glucose, and builds a strong neurological network.

But having higher dopamine from a slower COMT system also carries a disadvantage. When life becomes overly stressful, these COMT +/+ individuals will lose brain function as the level of catecholamines increases and falls off the right side of the bell curve.[5] Unfortunately, when the brain is flooded with catecholamines (on the right side of the bell curve), susceptibility to pain, anxiety, and even schizophrenia is increased.[6]

UNDERSTANDING THE DOPAMINE BELL CURVE

Though COMT SNPs can increase your focus and learning, they become a liability under high stress conditions because they cause dopamine to build up to toxic levels. Take a look at Figure 11.3. You can see three shapes placed along the curved line: COMT -/-, COMT +/-, and COMT +/+. These mark the different levels of frontal lobe dopamine found in individuals with different COMT genes.

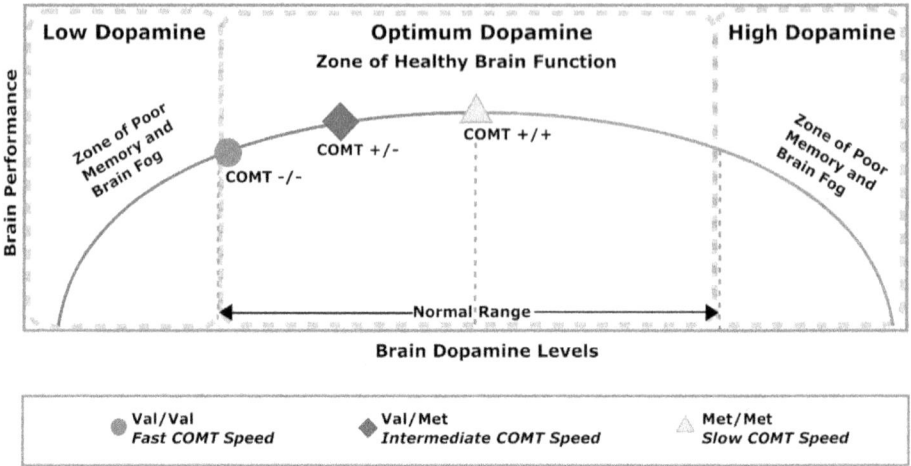

Figure 11.3 - Inverted U-shaped dopamine curve

The following list explains the differences between the different COMT gene patterns:

- **COMT V158M-/-** Fast Metabolizer. These individuals have a quicker COMT system, so they have lower levels of dopamine at a steady, resting state. They can handle multiple stressors at a single time better than COMT +/- or +/+.

- **COMT V158M +/-** Intermediate Metabolizer. These individuals live in the middle between a fast and slow COMT. Compared to the -/- group, they have a slower COMT system, so they have slightly higher levels of dopamine at a steady, resting state. They can handle less stress than the COMT **-/-** but more than the COMT +/+.

- **COMT V158M +/+** Slow Metabolizer. These individuals have the slowest COMT system, so they have the highest levels of dopamine at a steady, resting state. They have higher performance and more brain function in low stress states but will lose brain function as the number of stressors increases.

We know that brain function is a bell curve with dysfunction on either end. When people with COMT genes become overly stressed, they end up with too much dopamine in their frontal lobe. The excess catecholamine activity pushes the individual from the optimum middle range off the right side of the curve. Once someone has too much dopamine built up in their brain, it begins interfering with output of the frontal lobe. This causes a decrease in brain function, as you can see in Figures 11.2 and 11.3. Excess dopamine/catecholamine activity in the frontal lobe predisposes individuals to burnout, insomnia, pain, anxiety, worry, and in severe cases, schizophrenia and psychosis. We call individuals who experience this pattern the "high catecholamine phenotype," while we call individuals who suffer from the symptoms found on the left side of the curve the "low catecholamine phenotype."

To help clarify this point even further, consider a very interesting study that was published in 2012. In this study, researchers looked at brain function in rats, measuring how their brain function improved or worsened from different levels of adrenaline and glucose. Scientists discovered exactly what the catecholamine bell curve illustrates. They found that low levels of glucose and adrenaline slows brain function, that moderate levels optimized the brain (middle of the bell curve), and that high levels of these stimulants actually decreased brain function.[7] What we can take away from studies like this is that some stress is needed, but too much or too little will make your brain dysfunctional. And because the COMT (and MAO) gene is responsible for detoxifying adrenaline and dopamine, it has a big influence on this whole process. We all need some stress to get into the middle range, or sweet spot, of the bell curve, but too much stress pushes us literally over the edge.

Basically, when the body gets excessively stressed out, the COMT system cannot get rid of the adrenaline/dopamine/catecholamines fast enough. This makes the brain sick with too many toxic, inflammatory stress chemicals. When all those stress hormones are finished activating neurons, they must be detoxified. If the COMT enzyme is slowed, it will fall behind and won't be able to detoxify these neurotransmitters fast enough. Then the dopamine levels rise inside our brain and interfere with our normal brain function. This is why, all things being equal, the COMT +/+ gene predisposes us toward a phenotype of stress-induced illness.

Also, as the frontal lobe and neocortex become saturated with catecholamines, especially dopamine, the brain tries to protect itself from these potent chemicals by ignoring them. When our insulin is too high, we can get insulin resistance; when our cortisol is too high, we can get cortisol resistance; and we can develop *dopamine resistance* if dopamine levels rise too high as well. Studies show that when we release dopamine in high amounts, the brain reduces the number of dopamine receptors, effectively ignoring the dopamine signal altogether.[8] The body ignores constant stimuli, so it will do its best to ignore the excess dopamine and catecholamines. The end result is a constant roller coaster of depression, anxiety, fatigue, lack of focus, and brain fog that makes getting through the day a challenging proposition.

COMT DYSFUNCTION AND EMOTIONS

Emotional issues and imbalances are also very common in individuals with COMT SNPs. When the brain becomes less functional from stress, toxins, traumatic brain injury, or other factors, the result is a loss of emotional control. When the brain is healthy, it keeps our subconscious emotions and fears at bay. Without the neocortex and frontal lobe working well, our subconscious impulses can erupt and disrupt our behavior.

These emotional urges live in the limbic system. When the neocortex and frontal lobe are healthy, they keep the limbic system in a calm, resting state. However, when the neocortex isn't working well, the deeper emotional and fear-based programing in our limbic system begins to show up. These deeper emotional impulses may show up as anxiety, fear, worry, OCD behaviors, ADD, ADHD, and a host of other brain-based concerns.

You may know someone who has suffered a severe head injury and noticed their personality changed almost overnight. Head injuries can damage the neocortex and the frontal lobe of the brain, which makes the brain unable to control the urges and deeper emotional patterns from the limbic system. This is the same principal we see with COMT gene SNPs. Excess catecholamines can cause loss of frontal lobe function and lead to these behaviors. When you give children too much sugar and see their behavior degenerate as they lose self-control, you are watching the frontal lobe become overstimulated and dysfunctional. The same thing can happen in people with slow COMT genes when they get too much dopamine in their frontal lobe.

The brain really doesn't want EXTRA dopamine–like the Goldilocks character doesn't want the overly hot or cold porridge. The brain, like Goldilocks, wants the level of dopamine to be in the middle, the sweet spot, where brain function is optimized. And getting to the optimum "Goldilocks" level of dopamine is why it is so important to know how to balance catecholamine levels.

CATECHOLAMINE PHENOTYPES

What I am getting at by sharing all this information with you, both in this chapter and throughout this book, is that we need to understand the phenotype. We discussed the concept of phenotype back in chapter 3, but here the concept really comes into play. Once we know someone's phenotype (their genetic tendency plus the environment over time), the solution for their problem becomes clear. In other words, correctly identifying the phenotype is the first and most important step toward finding a lasting solution.

I often tell my patients that my job as the doctor is to identify their phenotype correctly. If we can do that, people are going to get better. To use all these amazing MTHFR-related SNPs and pathways correctly, I have to know if someone has a high catecholamine or low catecholamine phenotype. This is absolutely the most critical issue in helping my patients with methylation-gut-brain issues! Knowing which phenotype you have helps you decide which supplements, diets, and lifestyle changes are necessary.

The takeaway is that people tend to be in one category or the other–high or low catecholamines relative to serotonin. Low dopamine combined with low serotonin gives us feelings of depression. When adrenaline and/ or dopamine is raised because of stress, excitement, food, drugs, and the like, we can feel more of an anxiety situation. Low catecholamines plus low serotonin creates a grumpy, angry, "hangry" depression. When catechol- amines are raised but serotonin remains low, we get more of an anxiety, edgy, wired, and tired sort of experience. Again, it's not a perfect science, but it's close enough to get you moving in the right direction.

The following is exactly what I tell my patients to help them understand their phenotype. People sometimes don't fit nicely into either category, and this can confuse both doctor and patient. Despite the confusion, just remember that individuals will always have a dominant phenotype. Which- ever phenotype fits the best is the phenotype that needs to be treated.

High catecholamine explanation

Situations can arise inside the body that make it difficult for the body to de- toxify catecholamines such as dopamine, adrenaline, and norepinephrine. Genetic polymorphisms in the COMT gene, as well as bacterial phenols from the gut, can slow down the body's removal of adrenaline and dopa- mine. If your body makes something at a steady rate but doesn't remove it quickly, the levels inside can rise rapidly. This is what happens with high catecholamine phenotypes. These individuals are able to produce adren- aline and dopamine very quickly, but they lack the ability to clear it from their system fast enough. In these individuals, catecholamine levels build up fast and lead to anxiety, panic, worry, insomnia, chronic pain, and other frustrating health conditions.

Low catecholamine explanation

Many individuals with a tendency for lower catecholamines (dopamine, norepinephrine, epinephrine) will inadvertently seek out drugs, chemicals, or activities designed to raise dopamine and the catecholamines. These are forms of self-medication. It doesn't matter if we are binging on food, drugs, or exercise—the whole reason we feel compelled to perform those acts is that our brain is looking for something, anything, that can raise dopamine. When dopamine is low in individuals, they often experience anger, moodiness, grumpiness, compulsive behaviors, and high risk and addictive behaviors. Additionally, people with low catecholamines are excessively sleepy, even pseudo-narcoleptic, and take many naps, sleep long hours, and fall asleep easily. These are the most common signs and symptoms of low dopamine.

CONCLUSION

The issue of stress and how we react to it is greatly influenced by our genes. Many people are suffering in our culture with stress-related illnesses, and we need to do a better job of taking care of them. The problem with the COMT gene is how it alters the level of dopamine in the brain. The genetic root of depression, anxiety, pain, and insomnia lies in the COMT pathway because it determines how much dopamine and catecholamines are inside the nervous system.

The problem isn't that COMT +/+ people produce too much dopamine; the problem is that they don't detoxify dopamine and catecholamines very quickly. If your body makes something at a normal rate, but gets rid of it at a slowed rate, you'll likely end up with a high amount of that something in your body. In other words, if you have a problem detoxifying dopamine because of COMT +/+ genes, then you are going to struggle with the side effects of high dopamine. When you are under excessive stress, you are very likely going to have a problem with sleeping, pain, anxiety, panic, and worry.

The way to help people with COMT issues is to apply many of the concepts we have already discussed. Optimizing stomach function, removing phenols and aldehydes from the gut, treating oxalate issues, and other protocols all reduce the burden on the COMT system. Since we can't rearrange our genes, we need to take as much stress off our genetics as possible. In addition to the protocols for killing bugs, improving digestion, and supporting COMT pathways, COMT +/+ people need to avoid multiple stressors at the same time. This is the most important lifestyle recommendation I can make to people with COMT issues. If we follow the advice we've seen so far, we can change the environment inside the brain and dramatically improve quality of life. In the next and final chapter, I will discuss the last piece of this genius body puzzle: how our hormones influence the COMT system and cause stress and anxiety all by themselves.

HIGH AND LOW DOPAMINE PROTOCOL

Of all the discoveries I have made in the past 9 years, by far the most important one is the catecholamine bell curve. Dr. Robert Rakowski heavily influenced my thinking by teaching how all body systems work on a bell curve—being too fat or being too thin, drinking too much water or not drinking enough, eating too many calories or eating too few, etc. When we apply this bell curve concept to brain function, we can see that people either have high catecholamine or low catecholamine tendencies. The only question now is how do we fix it?

To fix the catecholamine bell curve is to balance the brain. People who are too low in dopamine need to increase the production of catecholamines. Those who have too much dopamine need ways to decrease production and/or speed up detoxification of catecholamines. The following protocols have helped me make headway and treat my patients' mood, anxiety, depression, and mental functions in ways that were impossible before we used this model.

RECOMMENDED LAB TESTING:

I recommend the Routine Blood Tests and the Organic Acid Test in appendix B for assessing the levels of catecholamines and serotonin-related compounds. To make full use of the information in this book, I recommend following the instructions found in appendix A to get your own detailed genetic report.

LOW CATECHOLAMINE PROTOCOL:

L-Tyrosine – 2 capsules 3 times per day with meals. Tyrosine is the required building block for both thyroid hormone and dopamine/adrenaline production.† (Nutridyn)

Methyl Complete – 2 capsules 2 times per day with meals. Therapeutic levels of methylB12, methylfolate, and other cofactors to increase BH4 and improve methylation.† (Nutridyn)

Stress Essentials Balance – 2 capsules between breakfast and lunch, and 2 capsules between lunch and dinner. Contains adaptogenic herbs that assist the body in producing higher levels of catecholamines.† (Nutridyn)

Dynamic Daily Meal – 1 scoop once or twice per day as a snack or meal replacement. High quality pea and rice protein helps to increase neurotransmitters and increase brain function.† (Nutridyn)

Pure D-Phenyl-Relief – 1 capsule 3 times per day with meals. Provides pharmaceutical grade D-Phenylalaline to support dopamine production.† (Nutridyn)

HIGH CATECHOLAMINE PHENOTYPE PROTOCOL:

Melatonin Liquid – 1 mg of melatonin every waking hour for 7 days. Then reduce the dose to 1 mg every 2 or 3 hours throughout the day, or take 1 mg every hour between dinner and bedtime. This product is to be taken at the top of every hour that you are awake. Take it from the time you wake in the morning until the time you fall asleep at night. If you happen to awaken at night, take another 1 mg and then go back to sleep. There is no need to wake up and take the melatonin when you sleep; if you are asleep, just keep sleeping and then start the melatonin every hour once you wake in the morning. Melatonin lowers cortisol release from the adrenal glands and reduces dopamine and catecholamine levels in the brain. The only known side effect of too much melatonin is being excessively groggy or sleepy.† (Nutridyn)

Liposomal L-Theanine – 100 mg of L-theanine (1-dropperfull) every waking hour for 7 days. Then reduce the dose to 100 mg every 2 or 3 hours throughout the day, or take 100 mg every hour between dinner and bedtime. This product is to be taken at the top of every hour that you are awake. Take it from the time you wake in the morning until the time you fall asleep at night. If you happen to awaken at night, take another 100 mg and then go back to sleep. There is no need to wake up and take the L-theanine when you sleep; if you are asleep, just keep sleeping and then start the L-theanine every hour once you wake in the morning. L-theanine is an amino acid from green tea that increases GABA, reduces glutamate, and lowers anxiety. It has been proven to lower cortisol and catecholamines in the brain.† (Nutridyn)

Niacinamide 500 – 1 to 2 capsules 2 times per day with meals. Provides high levels of niacinamide, which helps the body improve the detoxification of catecholamines.† (Nutridyn)

Magtein – 3 to 5 capsules 30 minutes before bedtime. Magnesium L-Threonate is able to cross the blood brain barrier more effectively than other forms of magnesium. It has a calming effect on the brain and nervous system by inhibiting glutamate, promoting relaxation, sleep, and focus.† (Nutridyn)

Stress Essentials Relax – 2 capsules 3 times per day with meals. Helps to increase catecholamine detoxification inside the liver by increasing the speed of the COMT enzyme and improving bile and glutathione production.† (Nutridyn)

Hemp CBD Oil – Dosing ranges from 10mg to 180mg per day. The best advice for finding the correct amount of CBD support is to increase the dose by 5mg each day. Start with 5mg 2 times per day and then increase the dose by 5mg per day. The goal is to saturate the body with CBD, and this may require a dose of only 15mg per day or it may require a much higher dose of 100–180mg per day.

Once the optimum dose is found, stay at this dose for 2 weeks. Then slowly reduce dosage by one serving size every 3 to 5 days. Continue reducing the dosage every 3 to 5 days and stop reducing further if symptoms come back. If symptoms return, increase the dose back up to the previous dose where symptoms were managed. This means you aren't ready to reduce the dose quite yet, so wait an additional 2 weeks before trying to lower the dosage further. Ultimately you will find an optimum dose for your long-term support that is less than you needed for the initial 2-week loading period. CBD oil is a new and exciting compound that has shown promise for numerous difficult chronic diseases, from epilepsy to cancer. CBD is useful for the high catecholamine person because it inhibits dopamine and glutamate release in the brain. There is no known level of toxicity, no known drug interactions, and the only side effect is getting too sleepy.† (Elixinol)

---

†This statement has not been evaluated by the FDA. This product is not intended to diagnose, treat, cure, or prevent any disease. The information provided in this book is intended for your general knowledge only and is not a substitute for professional medical advice or treatment for specific medical conditions. You should not use this information to diagnose or treat a health problem or disease without consulting with a qualified healthcare provider. Please consult your healthcare provider with any questions or concerns you may have regarding your condition. Never disregard professional medical advice or delay in seeking it because of something you have read in this book.

REFERENCES

1. Barnett, J.H., K. Xu, J. Heron, et al. Cognitive effects of genetic variation in monoamine neurotransmitter systems: A population-based study of COMT, MAOA, and 5HTTLPR. *American Journal of Medical Genetics Part B: Neuropsychiatric Genetics.* (2011) 156(2): 158-67.

2. Dauvilliers, Y., M. Tafti, H.P. Landolt. Catechol-O-methyltransferase, dopamine, and sleep-wake regulation. *Sleep medicine reviews.* (2015) 22: 47-53.

3. de la Mora, M.P., A. Gallegos-Cari, Y. Arizmendi-García, et al. Role of dopamine receptor mechanisms in the amygdaloid modulation of fear and anxiety: structural and functional analysis. *Progress in neurobiology.* (2010) 90(2): 198-216.

4. Pezze, M.A., J. Feldon. Mesolimbic dopaminergic pathways in fear conditioning. *Progress in neurobiology.* (2004) 74(5): 301--20.

5. Meyer-Lindenberg, A., D.R. Weinberger. Intermediate phenotypes and genetic mechanisms of psychiatric disorders. *Nature Reviews Neuroscience.* (2006) 7(10): 818-27.

6. NIH/National Institute of Mental Health. Gene Enhances Prefrontal Function At A Price. *ScienceDaily.* www.sciencedaily.com/releases/2003/05/030508074640.htm. Accessed January 22, 2017.

7. Jensen, C.J., F. Demol, R. Bauwens, et al. Astrocytic β2 Adrenergic Receptor Gene Deletion Affects Memory in Aged Mice. *PLoS One.* (2016) 11(10): e0164721.

8. Minowa, M.T., S.H. Lee, M.M. Mouradian. Autoregulation of the human D1A dopamine receptor gene by cAMP. *DNA and cell biology.* (1996) 15(9): 759-67.

12.

THE HORMONAL CAUSE
OF STRESS AND ANXIETY

You can never learn less, you can only learn more.

—R. Buckminster Fuller

Optimizing methylation pathways means going beyond just deciding how much B12 or folate you need. Seeking to optimize methylation pathways also means you must go beyond looking at MTHFR to see all the genes and biochemicals that are impacting your health. We cannot optimize genes without understanding how our sex hormones can impact our genetic pathways.

As we all know, the differences between men and women are more than just skin deep. Our differences exist on physical, genetic, emotional, and hormonal levels. In fact, our sex hormones are so powerful, they don't just change the size and shape of our bodies, they change how we respond to stress in our environment. An important thing about sex hormones is that not only do they influence how our bodies look, but they also influence our brains and behaviors! Sex hormones influence brain function by altering the body's COMT and MAO pathways.

OVERVIEW OF SEX HORMONES, COMT, AND MAO

Many of you have performed a genetic test and are aware of your COMT and MAO status. Some of you may have inherited COMT and MAO genes, which are slower than the normal or "wild-type" genes. At first blush, these genes might seem like they are going to ruin your life. But as you've heard many times already, the genes you inherit from your parents are not your destiny, only your tendency when under stress. As you know by now, the body's environment has the biggest impact on how genes influence our lives. With that in mind, let's look at how the hormonal environment shapes the body's genetic tendencies.

Women have higher estrogen levels, and men have higher testosterone levels; this fact cannot be disputed. What isn't as well known is how these two hormones impact the metabolism of our neurotransmitters by altering the speed of the COMT and MAO pathways. You will remember that the COMT breakdown of dopamine has a major influence on how we react to stress. So much of our mood, our focus, and our memory is dependent on the level of dopamine in our brain.

Studies show that sex hormones play a critical role in how much dopamine we have in our brain. Our sex hormones play a major role in this process because both estrogen and testosterone influence the speed of COMT and MAO. So, logically, it makes sense that, physiologically speaking, men and women may react to stress differently. Because sex hormones have such a strong influence on our COMT and MAO pathways, men and women have different COMT and MAO speeds, *even if their genes and SNPs are identical*. Regardless of what shows up on your MTHFRSupport Variant Report, no matter which COMT or MAO genes you inherit, the hormones in your body are going to slow down or speed up your genes. It's that whole environment plus genes idea.

In other words, our sex hormones have an epigenetic effect on the methylation of neurotransmitters that is occurring independently of our genetics, apart from our genotype. A woman can be born with a fast COMT -/- genotype and yet experience all the symptoms of someone who is COMT +/+ when she is estrogen-dominant. She experiences these symptoms not because of her genotype, but because the environment is interfering with her methylation pathways. Her estrogen-dominance has a larger influence than her genes because the environment rules the roost!

In my practice I have worked with hundreds of men and women eager to balance their methylation cycle, improve their digestion, and regain their health. What I have noticed is a consistent pattern where women report suffering from feelings of anxiety and worry more often than men. Men on the other hand report suffering from feelings of depression, grumpiness, and anger more often than women. This pattern has been consistent in patients of all different ages and walks of life, suggesting that the root cause is related to something unique to each sex – the sex hormones. As you will see below, the reason for these unique differences between men and women has everything to do with how our sex hormones influence COMT and MAO genes.

Because of recent research showing how sex hormones influence brain chemistry and methylation-related pathways, we have a new level of understanding why women and men react differently to stress. It has everything to do with how estrogen and testosterone influence the methylation and breakdown of neurotransmitters. Figure 12.1 shows how sex hormones interfere with key methylation pathways.

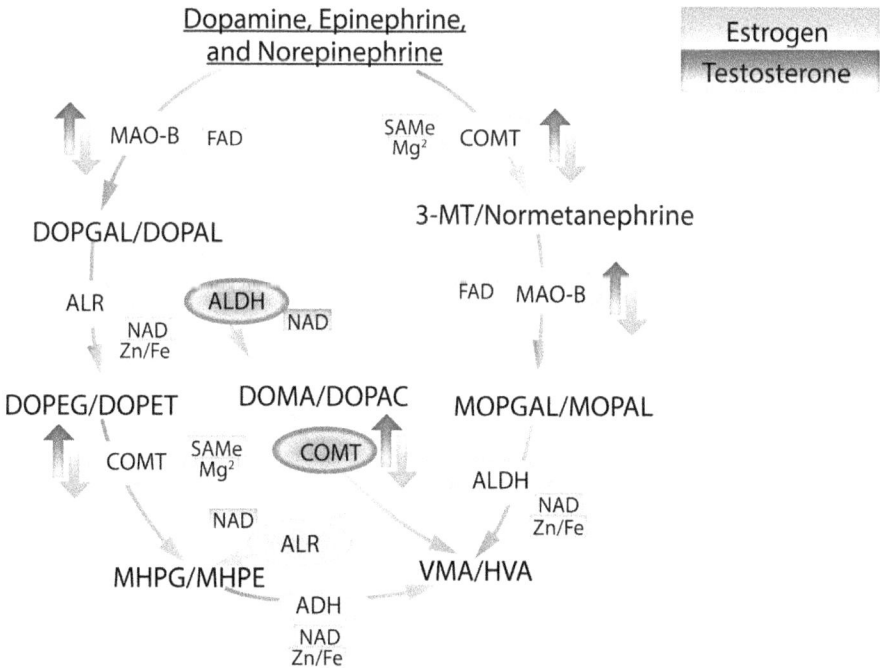

Figure 12.1 – *Down-arrows in pink mean the enzyme/gene is slowed down by estrogen; up-arrows in blue mean the enzyme/gene is sped up by testosterone.*

ESTROGEN, COMT, AND MAO

Compared to a healthy man, a healthy premenopausal woman should have much higher levels of estrogen and much lower levels of testosterone. This elevated estrogen is a natural consequence of being female and of having the ability to conceive children. In fact, when a woman becomes pregnant, her estrogen levels rise approximately 30-fold, providing the hormones her body needs to feed a growing baby. But that is only one type of estrogen, and in our environment estrogens come in many different flavors.

In addition to the estrogen made by the body, many women and men are exposed to toxic estrogens from chemicals such as birth control pills, heavy metals, fire retardants, BPA, and other sources, which increase the estrogen load. Many people are aware of the dangers of estrogenic toxins such as BPA, but fewer people know that pesticides, herbicides, and fire retardants act like estrogen as well. In fact, science has confirmed that heavy metals such as aluminum, arsenic, cadmium, lead, and mercury also activate estrogen receptors in our cells.[1] These metalloestrogens, as they are called, create yet another burden for our detoxification systems and alter our hormone balance even more. Ultimately, all this estrogen (both natural and man-made) causes problems for the COMT and MAO systems in the brain.

KEY CONCEPTS FOR COMT AND ESTROGEN

Estrogen is broken down by the COMT gene, a reaction that produces a calming, anti-cancer type of estrogen called 2-OH methoxy estrogen.[2] This estrogen is very important for health and helps prevent other symptoms of estrogen dominance such as PMS, clots and heavy bleeding, fibroids, endometriosis, and more. Without healthy levels of 2-OH estrogens, women have significant estrogen-dominance symptoms and are at an elevated risk of estrogen-related cancer. This is another reason why women need to make sure their COMT is working optimally.

Even though the COMT gene breaks down estrogen, it is also epigenetically slowed down by estrogen. Thus, the more estrogen a woman or man has, the slower their COMT system will be working. Highlighting this point, a research article from 2003 describes how hormonal therapy can be effective for dopamine-related diseases such as Parkinson's disease. Because estrogen slows COMT pathways, it may be of therapeutic value in Parkinson's patients who need a steady supply of dopamine in their brains.[3] Obviously, if more estrogen means more dopamine, it will benefit those who need more dopamine. Yet, if you already have too much dopamine, more estrogen is not the answer—it will make you have a low tolerance for stress!

Another review article published in 2015 shows how through environmental and epigenetic mechanisms, estrogen inhibits COMT pathways by about 30 percent. The researchers suggest that this is why many women have a predisposition toward a phenotype of high anxiety and a lower tolerance for stress.[4] So even if you aren't born with a SNP in your COMT pathway, just being female or having too much estrogen can make it feel like you do have a +/- or +/+ SNP.

In addition to the epigenetic effects that estrogen has on COMT pathways, it also greatly impacts the MAO system. Because estrogen impacts both COMT and MAO pathways, it is capable of having a major impact on the levels of frontal-lobe dopamine and stress hormones throughout the body. Research has clarified that a woman's mood is largely a reflection of how fast or slow her MAO-A system is working.

KEY CONCEPTS FOR MAO AND ESTROGEN

In a study from the 1970s, perimenopausal women with adrenal fatigue and depression were found to have a faster MAO system, leading to faster breakdown of dopamine and serotonin. When administered oral estrogen replacement, the women were relieved of their depression symptoms.[5] Menopause and adrenal fatigue both lower estrogen levels, so oral estrogen therapy helped slow down the MAO system, enabling the women to benefit from increased neurotransmitter levels. Although many women have too much estrogen and too much anxiety, women can experience the opposite problem of depression when their estrogen levels drop too low.

Interestingly, another study published in 2015 showed that post-partum depression is caused by a surge in the expression of MAO-A. Immediately after delivering a baby, a woman's body goes through a profound decline in estrogen. This rapid loss of estrogen, no longer necessary since pregnancy has ended, causes a reflexive increase in the speed of MAO-A.[6] As MAO-A speeds up, it detoxifies neurotransmitters much faster, leading to depression and other signs of post-partum depression such as apathy and excessive crying.

ESTROGEN CAUSES HIGH CATECHOLAMINE SYMPTOMS

If you are born with or are exposed to more estrogen in your body (both natural and man-made), you will tend to have more dopamine in your brain because your COMT/MAO pathway has been slowed. This elevation of dopamine and catecholamines makes you much more likely to experience anxiety, worry, insomnia, chronic pain, and other high catecholamine symptoms associated with a slow COMT/MAO system. A person with too much estrogen may wake up and feel confused why he or she cannot handle stress well at all. What this individual likely doesn't understand is how excess estrogen slows down their COMT and MAO systems, making them more sensitive to stress. The close relationship between estrogen and anxiety is shown in Figure 12.2.

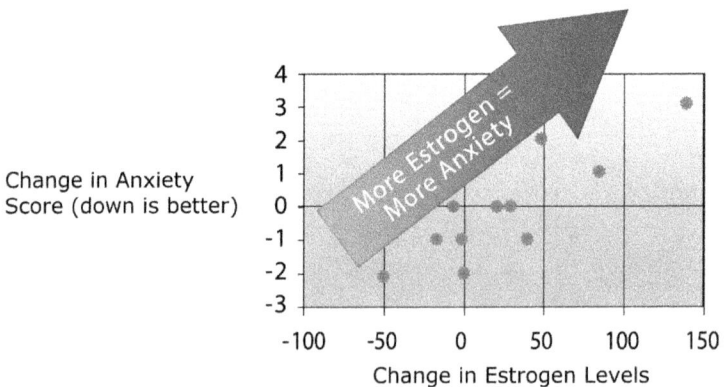

Figure 12.2 - *Studies prove that the more estrogen we have inside our bodies, the more anxiety we experience.*

An older study published in 1995 confirms the relationship between estrogen levels and MAO pathways. When analyzing the effects of sex hormones, researchers found that estrogen inhibited the MAO pathway in brain cells.[7] They concluded that this inhibition, this slowing down of the MAO system, was how estrogen creates its antidepressant effect. Remember the catecholamine bell curve from the last chapter: if estrogen can act as an antidepressant when dopamine is low, it can cause anxiety when dopamine is already too high to begin with. Like everything else in life, estrogen levels need to be balanced, or modulated, to avoid these two extremes.

These studies help to explain scientifically why women have a tendency toward anxiety and worry—more estrogen leads to more dopamine, adrenaline, and catecholamines in the brain. Estrogen has an antidepressant effect, but too much of it can cause a person to be unable to relax and calm down, and too little can lead to excessive depression. Because of this, estrogen balance is essential for women (and men) to experience their full potential. Of course, there are many facets to the estrogen story, and we are focusing on only one important part. To give you a visual of the bigger picture, Figure 12.3 illustrates the many problems associated with unbalanced estrogen levels:

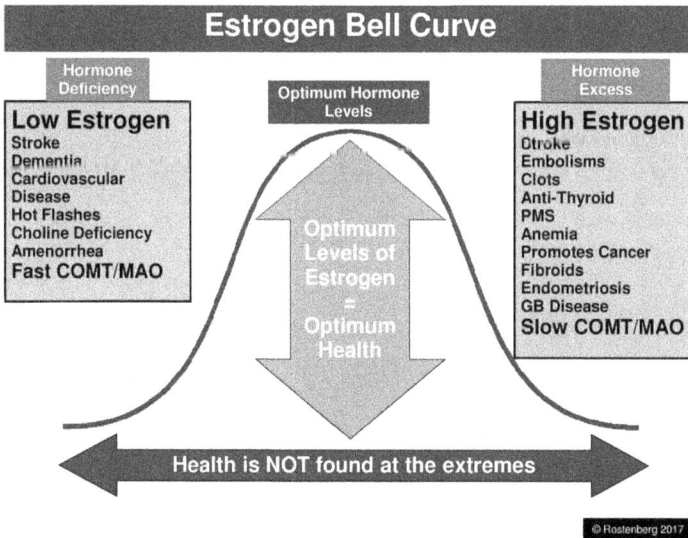

Figure 12.3 - *Bell curve showing reduced COMT/ MAO activity with elevated levels of estrogen*

You can see how estrogen dominance, by slowing down COMT and MAO, will make it more difficult for us to deal with stressful life situations such as a new job, new child, new relationship, relocating to a new town, and others. Excess estrogen will literally slow down our methylation pathways, making us less able to tolerate increased stress. And as estrogen does one thing, testosterone will probably do the opposite. Let's take a look at the testosterone research to see if that holds true.

TESTOSTERONE, COMT, AND MAO

In terms of the COMT and MAO pathways, the male sex hormone testosterone has the opposite effect of estrogen. Testosterone increases the genetic expression of COMT and MAO enzymes in the body, leading to lower levels of dopamine, norepinephrine, and epinephrine. If you are a man with healthy levels of testosterone in your body, you will tend to have a deficit of dopamine, because your COMT and MAO enzymes are going faster. This means men gravitate toward activities that raise the catecholamine neurotransmitters, since these chemicals will help balance the brain and have a calming, soothing effect on the nervous system.

For many men, doing things labeled "stressful" or "risky" actually helps to balance their brain function. This is why men tend to feel relaxed after going to the shooting range, attending a martial arts class, or riding a motorcycle at high speeds. Since men are supposed to have higher testosterone and lower estrogen, they tend to need more adrenaline in their life to feel balanced and calm. Many men are drawn to things that are dangerous because these activities raise catecholamines, dopamine, and adrenaline. And when you become aware of how testosterone impacts brain function, you will understand why.

KEY CONCEPTS FOR COMT, MAO, AND TESTOSTERONE

A study published in 2014 highlights how androgens such as testosterone and DHT increase the speed of the MAO and COMT pathways in the midbrain area, where much of our brain dopamine is produced.[8] Basically, the higher the testosterone levels in a man's body, the faster his body will detoxify catecholamines. Because men tend to break down dopamine and norepinephrine faster, they have developed an attraction for activities that are guaranteed to increase those neurochemicals. It is a form of self-medication that drives some men toward activities that are inherently risky.

Some men (as do some women) have a tendency for high risk behavior because it is an effective way to raise dopamine. Once you understand how testosterone drives dopamine levels down by speeding up COMT and MAO, it's obvious that much of what men do is designed to raise it back up. Men behave differently from women, and on some level, they are compelled to do so physiologically. To ward off depression, men seek activities that help move them into the middle of the catecholamine bell curve.

In some sense, risky activities of all kinds—be they motor racing, mountaineering, climbing, surfing, cage fighting, entrepreneurship, etc.—act like a drug. They increase dopamine in the brain similar to heroin, cocaine, and nicotine. The dopamine we get from taking risks is always the same, but the side effects of activities are different. Obviously, the side effect of crashing your motorcycle or falling off a mountain are different from the side effects of being addicted to heroin or cocaine. Choosing the side effect is more important than choosing the drug. The dopamine you get is always the same, but the side effects can either enrich or destroy your life—so choose wisely!

Finally, not everything that testosterone does to our brain impacts COMT and MAO. Some effects of testosterone simply help offset the negative impacts of estrogen. A study from 2012 showed that testosterone increases the brain's expression of estrogen receptor beta—the protective, calming type of estrogen receptor.[9] Estrogen receptor beta (ER beta) is an important part of our hormone system, because it helps to protect tissues such as the breasts, ovaries, uterus, and prostate from the toxic effects of estrogens.

ER beta acts like a toxic estrogen antidote in many tissues, including the brain. When testosterone upregulates this important receptor, it is helping to reduce the negative effects of high estrogen for both men and women. It is another small environmental factor that, when combined with everything else we've covered, helps us see the importance of balancing our sex hormones.

CONCLUSION

What I see every day in my clinic is that estrogen dominance, toxins, and hormone imbalances are major causes of anxiety in both men and women. This fact doesn't make sense until you understand how estrogen slows down the COMT and MAO pathways, while testosterone speeds them up. Whether it results from adrenal fatigue, birth control pills, hormone replacement, chemical toxins, or other factors, estrogen dominance tends to cause imbalances in the brain and the methylation cycle. This also helps to explain why men and women deal with and react to stress so differently.

Although it is always refreshing to be able to explain why things happen, our work doesn't end here. The ultimate goal in helping our fellow humans is to provide solutions that have a lasting, life-changing impact. Understanding how hormones change the levels of catecholamines in our brain might be the most important fact I have shared with you in this whole book—and they might deserve a book of their own someday.

Applying the ideas in this chapter may change your life or the life of a patient in ways they never thought possible. You've now got the tools required to not only see a list of symptoms, but to hear the body tell you a story about its genes and the environment within. Combined with the information I've already given you in previous chapters, the hormonal component to why we feel stress and anxiety is the final piece of this genius body puzzle. Take it, run with it, and let me know how it works for you!

ESTROGEN AND TESTOSTERONE PROTOCOL

Before you start working on your hormones, you should ensure that your gut and digestive system are optimized using the protocols I've shared with you in previous chapters. You should know how to balance your blood sugar and have a good idea whether you are a high catecholamine or low catecholamine phenotype. Once you have a handle on these concepts, you can begin to balance your hormones with the protocols described here.

The diet choices we make can have a large influence on our hormonal health. Entire books are written to explain the benefits of various diets, so I won't get into much detail here. Basically, my only advice is to make sure you are avoiding xenoestrogens (artificial estrogens) in the food supply by eating organic dairy, butter, and meat. Avoiding conventionally raised meat, eggs, and dairy will help you avoid some of the worst toxic estrogens in the food supply. Also, it is important to eat local and organic food as much as possible. GMO and conventionally grown fruits and veggies have an enormous toxin load and should be avoided if possible.

Most of the toxins—herbicides, pesticides, and fungicides—used in farming act like estrogens inside our bodies. How can you have hormone balance if your body is constantly exposed to artificial hormones from your food? If your goal is hormone balance, you should be committed to purchasing and/or growing the best food possible.

RECOMMENDED LAB TESTING:

I recommend the Routine Blood Tests and the DUTCH hormone test in appendix B for assessing the levels of estrogen, testosterone, and other sex hormones. To make full use of the information in this book, I recommend following the instructions found in appendix A to get your own detailed genetic report.

HIGH ESTROGEN / ESTROGEN DOMINANCE PROTOCOL:

Dynamic Hormone Balance – 1 scoop 2 times per day for 30 or more days. Once symptoms improve, reduce the dose to 2 scoops 2 times per day for only the 7 days preceding menstruation. For example, if your cycle is 28 days long, this means you would drink 2 shakes per day on days 22-28, and then stop when your cycle begins. Repeat this each month if necessary. Dynamic Hormone Balance gives the body extra support for detoxifying estrogen and helping to convert estrogen in the calming and protective 2-OH estrogen. Dynamic Hormone

Balance can be used on an ongoing basis to support healthy estrogen metabolism.† (Nutridyn)

Estro Balance– 2 capsules 2 times per day with meals. Provides the same estrogen-balance and detox-supporting nutrition as Dynamic Hormone Balance but in a tablet instead of a powder. Provides methylation support and phytoestrogen extracts to improve estrogen detoxification through the 2-OH pathway.† (Nutridyn)

Myo-Inositol Complex – 6 capsules per day. This versatile supplement contains myo-inositol, which improves insulin resistance, helping to decrease testosterone and balance female hormones. This product has been used successfully to treat polycystic ovary syndrome (PCOS), and it helps women regulate their cycle.† (Nutridyn)

I-3-C Plus – 1 capsule 3 times per day with meals. Contains the active ingredient Indole-3-Carbinol from the cruciferous vegetable family. This compound contains DIM and aids the liver in creating healthy 2-OH estrogens, reducing estrogen dominance.† (Nutridyn)

Chasteberry – 1 capsule 2 times per day with meals. Provides herbal support for progesterone production which helps alleviate symptoms of PMS and estrogen dominance.† (Nutridyn)

LOW TESTOSTERONE PROTOCOL:

Dynamic Hormone Balance – 1 scoop 2 times per day for 30 or more days. Though this product was designed originally to treat women, it has proven to be an excellent tool for men as well. The brain considers estrogen to be equivalent to testosterone; meaning the brain doesn't care if we have high estrogen or high testosterone. The only thing the brain cares about is the overall level of sex hormones. If a man has high estrogen, his brain stops telling his testes to produce testosterone because, from the brain's point of view, there is plenty of hormone. The way around this for men is to detoxify estrogen. When men remove excess estrogen from their bodies, they begin to trigger the production of testosterone. Because Dynamic Hormone Balance is so effective at helping our bodies remove estrogen, it is a great method for men to raise their testosterone naturally.† (Nutridyn)

Testro Balance – 2 capsules 2 times per day with meals. Provides broad-spectrum testosterone support by inhibiting aromatase and supporting the healthy detoxification of estrogen through the liver's 2-OH pathway.† (Nutridyn)

Omega Pure DHA 600 – 2 softgels 2 times per day with meals. DHA is a key Omega-3 fatty acid that is found in high concentrations in the testes. Sperm quality and testosterone levels are greatly improved by dietary intake of DHA.† (Nutridyn)

His Vitality – 1 capsule 2 times per day with meals. Contains herbal support for healthy male sexual function, libido, stress resilience, and vitality.† (Nutridyn)

---

†This statement has not been evaluated by the FDA. This product is not intended to diagnose, treat, cure, or prevent any disease. The information provided in this book is intended for your general knowledge only and is not a substitute for professional medical advice or treatment for specific medical conditions. You should not use this information to diagnose or treat a health problem or disease without consulting with a qualified healthcare provider. Please consult your healthcare provider with any questions or concerns you may have regarding your condition. Never disregard professional medical advice or delay in seeking it because of something you have read in this book.

REFERENCES

1. Darbre, P.D. Metalloestrogens: an emerging class of inorganic xenoestrogens with potential to add to the oestrogenic burden of the human breast. *J Appl Toxicol.* (2006) 26(3): 191-7.

2. Tal, R. The role of hypoxia and hypoxia-inducible factor-1alpha in preeclampsia pathogenesis. *Biol Reprod.* (2012) 87(6): 134.

3. Jiang, H., T. Xie, D.B. Ramsden, et al. Human catechol-O-methyltransferase down-regulation by estradiol. *Neuropharmacology.* (2003) 45(7): 1011-18.

4. Dauvilliers,Y., M. Tafti, H.P. Landolt. Catechol-O-methyltransferase, dopamine, and sleep-wake regulation. *Sleep Med Rev.* (2015) 22: 47-53.

5. Klaiber, E.L., D.M. Broverman, W. Vogel, et al. Effects of estrogen therapy on plasma MAO activity and EEG driving responses of depressed women. *Am J Psychiatry.* (1972) 128(12): 1492-8.

6. Sacher, J., P.V. Rekkas, A.A. Wilson, et al. Relationship of monoamine oxidase-A distribution volume to postpartum depression and postpartum crying. *Neuropsychopharmacology.* (2015) 40(2): 429-35.

7. Ma, Z.Q., E. Violani, F. Villa, et al. Estrogenic control of monoamine oxidase A activity in human neuroblastoma cells expressing physiological concentrations of estrogen receptor. *Eur J Pharmacol.* (1995) 284(1-2): 171-6.

8. Godar, S.C., M. Bortolato. Gene-sex interactions in schizophrenia: focus on dopamine neurotransmission. *Front Behav Neurosci.* (2014) 8: 71.

9. Purves-Tyson, T.D., D.J. Handelsman, K.L. Double, et al. Testosterone regulation of sex steroid-related mRNAs and dopamine-related mRNAs in adolescent male rat substantia nigra. *BMC Neurosci.* (2012) 13: 95.

APPENDIX A

DNA AND METHYLATION GENE TESTING

This appendix covers my advice for genetic testing. Many of you might already know about the recent advances in genetic testing, while others reading this may need some more information. In general, you test your genetics through saliva testing. For the cost of a single genetic blood test, you can obtain a report covering thousands upon thousands of important genes. It is a no-brainer!

The two companies I recommend are 23andMe and AncestryDNA. Although there are new companies popping up all the time, I can vouch for the accuracy and usefulness of these two companies. My advice would be to compare prices (AncestryDNA is usually significantly less expensive) and choose the one you like best. Consider using a fake name when submitting your DNA data. It is your right to privacy, and in our ultra-connected world, you should place at least some barriers between your sensitive personal data and those who want to exploit it. Fake names will keep your DNA data somewhat anonymous, protecting your privacy.

Both 23andMe and AncestryDNA analyze your saliva sample and provide insights into your family, health, and other genetic information. Though that info can be interesting, it isn't what you really need to understand your genetics. To learn about your COMT, MTHFR, MAO, SULT, SNPs, etc., you need what is called the "Raw Data" file, which is used to generate an easy-to-read report. It will be available to you once your saliva sample has been processed and your DNA results are ready to view. Each company will allow you to download this Raw Data file to your desktop, and from there you have to perform one more step.

Once your Raw Data file has been downloaded, go to the website MTH-FRSupport.com and order the Variant Report, a handy tool that organizes the complicated genotype data into an easy-to-read format. The colorful Variant Report you can download from MTHFRSupport offers the best chance of understanding your genetics. Sterling Hill, owner of MTHFRSupport, is constantly updating her report, making it the most state-of-the-art product available.

This report lists whether or not you inherited the "good, bad, or ugly" version of a gene. It categorizes genes and assigns them colors such as green, yellow, and red for easy identification and learning. Sterling's Variant Report saves time and simplifies things, which comes in handy for obvious reasons. Figure A.1 shows an MTHFRSupport Variant Report, showing green, yellow, and red SNPs. This is the best tool available for deciphering the complexities of your genetic information.

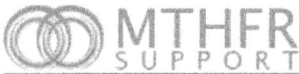

MTHFRSupport Variant Report v2.4
Based on: Test Data
http://www.mthfrsupport.com

SNP ID	SNP Name	Risk Allele	Your Alleles	Your Results
	Liver Detox - Phase I (Figure 1)			
rs1048943	CYP1A1*2C A4889G	C	TT	-/-
rs1799814	CYP1A1*4 C2453A	T	GG	-/-
rs2472304	CYP1A2*1F	A	AA	+/+
rs762551	CYP1A2*1F C164A	C	AA	-/-
rs2069526	CYP1A2*1K -739T>G	G	TT	-/-
rs56276455	CYP1A2*3 D348N	A	GG	-/-
rs28399424	CYP1A2*6 R431W	T	CC	-/-
rs28936700	CYP1B1 10233C>T	T	CC	-/-
rs1056827	CYP1B1 A119S	A	AA	+/+
rs1056836	CYP1B1 L432V	C	GG	-/-
rs1800440	CYP1B1 N453S	T	TT	+/+
rs10012	CYP1B1 R48G	G	GG	+/+
rs9282671	CYP1B1 T241A	A	AA	+/+
rs5031016	CYP2A6 T1412C	G	AA	-/-
rs28399454	CYP2A6 V365M	T	CC	-/-
rs1801272	CYP2A6*2 A1799T	T	AA	-/-
rs35303484	CYP2B6 A136G	G	AA	-/-
rs34097093	CYP2B6 C1132T	T	CC	-/-
rs8192719	CYP2B6 C26570T	T	CT	+/-
rs28399499	CYP2B6 I328T	C	TT	-/-
rs3745274	CYP2B6 Q172H	T	GT	+/-
rs8192709	CYP2B6 R22C	T	CC	-/-
rs3211371	CYP2B6 R487C	T	CC	-/-
rs1042389	CYP2B6 T1421C	C	TT	-/-

Figure A.1 - *This is the easiest way to read your genotype. It is a sample taken from a variant report produced by Sterling Hill's MTHFRSupport application.*

Once you have this report in hand, you can start to work to unravel your genetic imbalances. I suggest working with a practitioner who has experience in this area, to avoid confusion and poor results. You may have a trusted doctor to work with, or you can search for a doctor near you on Sterling Hill's website under the "Find a Practitioner" tab. Or you may want to be one of the thousands of patients who work with our Boise office directly. You can contact my office directly via email at care@redmountainclinic.com or via phone at 208-322-7755 to begin the process of getting care through our clinic.

One final note for those of you who are apprehensive about looking at your own genetic report: Learning about your own genotype and family history is very exciting, but a word of caution is necessary. Several companies provide genotype reports based on your genes that estimate your likelihood of disease. This tends to ignore the scientific fact that the environment, the epigenetics around the cell, actually controls our genes—not the genes themselves. Philosophically and scientifically, I take issue with reports that tell people they have a "X percent" risk of cancer, or heart disease, or depression. It turns people into victims and isn't accurate.

Consider that research published by the Mayo Clinic in 2016 shows that only 3 percent of the US adult population has a healthy lifestyle.[1] So how can we blame a gene for causing disease, when 97 percent of the population has a lifestyle that makes them sick? That is muddying the water and blaming our ancestors instead of our choices. According to Bruce Lipton, PhD, and other leaders in the field, only 5 percent of diseases can be blamed on genetics. Do yourself a favor and pay small attention to the disease risk in your genetic genotype report. Scientifically, the only real risk we know about is our lifestyle, and that is something you have 100 percent control over!

[1] Loprinzi, P.D., A. Branscum, J. Hanks, et al. Healthy lifestyle characteristics and their joint association with cardiovascular disease biomarkers in US adults. In *Mayo Clinic Proceedings*, 91(4). Elsevier (2016): 432-42.

APPENDIX B:

———

LABORATORY TESTING INFORMATION

In this section, you will find the tests I most often recommend to my patients. There are thousands of different blood, stool, urine, saliva, and other tests available through doctors and hospitals. We do not need to test everything under the sun; we just need to focus on what tests are required to help us find the root cause of our health problems. Every test has some value, but testing is very expensive, especially for individuals like my patients who pay out of pocket, so we try to focus on the most useful tests only.

The following list shows the tests we most often use in our office. On occasion, we have to branch out from these tests, but for more than 95 percent of our patients, these are the tests we use to help them regain their health and optimize their well-being. The most useful test by far is the Organic Acid Test, followed by the routine blood tests and then the DUTCH hormone test. Of course, we select different tests depending on the symptoms and complexity of each individual. I am providing a brief overview of these tests for you here, so you will have a reference as to which tests are most useful to you in your quest for optimizing your life and your health.

ORGANIC ACID TEST (OAT)

The Organic Acid Test (OAT) is an incredibly useful tool. The OAT is a urine test that is run through a complex chemical analysis to evaluate the levels of 75 individual molecules. Basically, the OAT is testing your urine for volatile organic compounds, or VOCs, just like the VOCs that were once present in paint. The OAT can tell you a great deal about your chronic health issue. I like the OAT specifically because it helps me answer the following questions:

- How much yeast and bacteria are in your body?

- What species of yeast and bacteria are present?

- How many oxalates are in your body?

- Do you have high or low catecholamines?

- Do you have high or low serotonin?

- Do you have enough methylation occurring in your cells?

- Are you high or low in B vitamins, antioxidants, glutathione, etc.?

- Is your body able to burn fat for fuel?

- Are your mitochondria strong, or weak and inefficient?

Over the past 3 years, I have seen more than 500 OAT results from my patients, and it has been an incredible asset. It enables us to connect the dots between your gut, your brain, your mitochondria, and your genetics like no other test in existence. Obviously, if you want to use all the cutting-edge information found in *Your Genius Body*, you need a high-quality test like the OAT to get you started.

The OAT I recommend is provided only through Great Plains Laboratory (800-288-0383, www.greatplainslaboratory.com). Other companies offer an "organic acid test" but they omit oxalate testing and also have fewer yeast (aldehyde) and bacterial (phenol) markers. Suffice it to say, you are better off spending your resources on the Great Plains Test as it is the most useful OAT on the market.

The cost for this test is still $309 as of fall 2017. Some insurance plans cover this test (make sure to ask Great Plains Laboratory for details), so it could be even less expensive for some of you. For anyone with a chronic health problem whose doctors are scratching their heads, the OAT from Great Plains Laboratory should be at the top of your list for testing.

ROUTINE BLOOD TESTS

Many of you will be familiar with some or all of these tests. I would call these lab tests "routine" in that they should be done from time to time. Nothing fancy here—just good ol' preventative medicine. They help to make sure all the major metabolic systems in your body—liver, kidney, immune, methylation, blood sugar, adrenal, pancreas, etc.—are being properly supported. I would recommend they be performed on a yearly basis to monitor health and progress regardless of the diagnosis or label you have been given.

The blood lab tests I recommend for my patients include the following:

- CBC with differential

- Comprehensive metabolic panel

- Ferritin

- HgA1C

- Homocysteine

- hs-CRP

- Insulin

- Iron

- Lipid panel

- Erythrocyte sedimentation rate

- TIBC

- Vitamin D 25-OH

These tests are performed together first thing in the morning, after fasting approximately 12 hours. (Fasting is required only for the comprehensive metabolic panel, lipid panel, and the insulin, but since we usually do them all together, we include the fasting instructions to our patients). These tests are very common and should be available through any hospital, medical doctor, or lab company such as Quest or LabCorp.

CHRONIC VIRUS BLOOD TESTS

Sometimes routine blood tests and OAT are not enough by themselves. In many cases of patients with chronic fatigue, fibromyalgia, adrenal weakness, and brain fog, there is evidence of viral involvement. In other words, many people with chronic health issues are actually suffering from an unrecognized and untreated virus infection. Virus infections can persist under the radar for weeks, months, or even years if our immune system is not able to address the infection adequately. In many chronically ill and chronically stressed patients, the immune system is operating far below 100 percent, making chronic virus issues more common.

Viruses replicate by putting their DNA inside our DNA. When infected with a virus, the viral DNA actually hijacks our own cellular machinery, forcing our cells to make more copies of the virus. Instead of making proteins and molecules to help us heal, the virus directs the cells to reproduce more invaders. We discussed in chapter 3 how our body uses methyl groups to regulate genes, and to repress them and turn them off. When our genes are methylated, they get a carbon atom with three hydrogens stuck on top of them and they are turned off. Since we know viruses insert themselves into our own DNA, the viral DNA acts just like a gene—it can either be silenced or expressed via the methylation process.

My opinion is that people with MTHFR and methylation-related issues are more susceptible to chronic viruses because they are less able to methylate fully and turn off the viral DNA inside their cells. And there truly is a lot of viral DNA inside our cells. Recent research suggests that 40 percent of our human DNA is "parasitic" residue left behind by viruses either we or our ancestors encountered! If your methylation is weak, and you had mononucleosis in eighth grade, it can come back 20 years later during periods of high stress. The way to make sure you do not have a chronic virus is to do the testing listed here.

Blood tests for chronic virus infection include EBV, HSV-1, HSV-2, VZV, and

CMV. You want to test the IgM and IgG levels for all these viruses. These tests are also available through any hospital, medical doctor, or lab company such as Quest or LabCorp.

CHRONIC VIRUS PROTOCOL:

In addition to taking L-Lysine and B6 from chapter 5, I recommend the following supplements whenever patients uncover a hidden or chronic viral infection:

Ganoderma Plus - 2 capsules 3 times per day. Ganoderma spore powder is a highly concentrated extract of Reishi mushroom. This plant helps increase white blood cell function and has proven very effective for helping the body get rid of chronic viral infections.† (Nutridyn)

L-Glutamine Powder - 2 tablespoons 3 times per day with or without meals. Glutamine helps to increase the total number of white blood cells; it helps our white blood cells do a better job of clearing infections.† (Nutridyn)

Immune Support - 1 tablet per day with or without meals. Provides broad-spectrum nutrients to assist the white blood cell function, increase glutathione, and help clear viruses.† (Nutridyn)

I have one last thing to mention regarding viral IgM and IgG tests. There is some confusion in the medical system about what a positive test means. Any positive result on these viral blood tests indicates an active infection. If your test comes back and either one or both of your IgG or IgM levels are elevated for any virus, it means you are in the process of fighting it.

---

†This statement has not been evaluated by the FDA. This product is not intended to diagnose, treat, cure, or prevent any disease. The information provided in this book is intended for your general knowledge only and is not a substitute for professional medical advice or treatment for specific medical conditions. You should not use this information to diagnose or treat a health problem or disease without consulting with a qualified healthcare provider. Please consult your healthcare provider with any questions or concerns you may have regarding your condition. Never disregard professional medical advice or delay in seeking it because of something you have read in this book.

An infection that happened 20 years ago will have undetectable levels of IgG and IgM. The reason for this is in the half-lives of IgG and IgM. These molecules at most have a half-life of around 20 days, which means approximately 3 months after you got over mono, for example, the test should come back normal. If you still have elevated viral antibodies weeks, months, or years since you had the illness, it indicates the virus has reactivated. Don't worry though, because you can use natural medicine tools to assist your immune system and optimize your methylation cycle so this problem is taken care of once and for all. Contact our office for a consultation and we can help you with a personalized virus-killing protocol.

COMPREHENSIVE STOOL TEST

Comprehensive Diagnostic Stool Testing involves sending in a sample of your stool to a laboratory for analysis. Normally for gut health, I use the OAT because it provides information about yeast and bacteria, and this is usually enough in most cases. When the OAT doesn't provide enough detail about the gut environment, my next favorite tool is to use a stool test. This type of testing detects the presence and species of pathogenic microorganisms such as yeast, parasites, and bacteria that contribute to chronic illness and neurological dysfunction. Where the OAT will tell you if you have high phenols and/or aldehydes, etc., the stool test will directly identify which specific pathogens are in your GI tract. Obviously, this is helpful information for many who have a chronic intestinal problem that has resisted routine treatments. In addition, this test provides helpful information about prescription and natural products effective against specific strains detected in the sample. The test also evaluates beneficial bacteria levels, intestinal immune function, overall intestinal health, and inflammation markers.

Because most of my patients are working with us out-of-pocket, we simply don't go overboard on testing. That said, sometimes a stool test is very useful; it is up to you and your doctor to decide whether the test is right for you. My favorite lab for performing stool testing is the GI Map test from Diagnostic Solutions Laboratory (877-485-5336, diagnosticsolutionslab.com).

DUTCH HORMONE TEST

One of the newest tests available for understanding your hormones is a dried urine test. The Dried Urine Test for Comprehensive Hormones, or DUTCH test, has become a valuable tool in my office for helping patients. As many of you are aware, there are several methods for hormone testing, and they all have some value. Blood tests are still used as the primary method of hormone testing by our medical system, and they accurately reflect the levels of hormone in the blood stream. Saliva testing is the next method many are familiar with. Saliva has the advantage of measuring the amount of the hormone that gets into your cells, which is more accurate than which levels are in the blood. But neither of these tests give you nearly the information found with the DUTCH.

What sets this test apart is how thorough it is in measuring your body's hormone system. The DUTCH test will measure not only your sex hormones—progesterone, testosterone, DHEA, and estrogen—but it will also measure several adrenal stress markers as well. The DUTCH test measures a total of 35 different hormones, which is by far the most in-depth test available. But that isn't even the best part. Not only does it measure the three different estrogens (estrone, estradiol, and estriol) as they circulate through your body, it also measures the estrogen metabolites that come from the detoxification process in the liver. In other words, the DUTCH test gives you instant feedback on how well you are detoxifying the estrogen-related hormones through the phase I and phase II systems. It shows who is at a greater risk for estrogen-related cancers due to an excess of 4-OH and 16-OH estrogen metabolites.

This test helps me identify which patients are at risk of hormone-related health problems; it shows me who needs methylation support and who needs support for improved estrogen-related detoxification. I recommend the DUTCH test because it is affordable, easy to collect, and provides data that no other testing method can.

To order this test, contact Precision Analytics (503-687-2050, https://dutchtest.com/shop/) and select the DUTCH Complete test kit. This test kit costs $399 as of fall 2017, and to my knowledge is not covered by insurance plans. However, we are able to offer this exact test to our patients for only $250. The difference almost covers the cost of a new patient consultation so it makes sense to reach out to our office and get on our schedule!

SIBO BREATH TEST

The gold standard test available for detecting SIBO is called the Lactulose Breath Test. Basically, you drink a highly fermentable liquid and then measure the increase in methane and hydrogen-sulfide gas over the next 2 or 3 hours. Most tests use a 2-hour measure, but some new tests now offer a 3-hour sample. This test is usually performed in a doctor's office, where you exhale multiple times into a special sealed container and send that to the lab. I usually diagnose SIBO by symptoms and by looking at the OAT results. However, there have been cases where OAT results were fine but the patient still had a strong case of SIBO, so the correlation isn't 100 percent. Like any test, use the SIBO breath test as a way to confirm your suspicions and justify major changes to your diet, lifestyle, supplements, etc. Before you make major changes to your life, it helps to have a test that confirms that you indeed have a problem.

Many labs offer this testing. We use Genova Diagnostics (800-522-4762, www.gdx.net) for the Lactulose SIBO Breath Test. The cost for this SIBO testing is usually between $100 and $200.

SULFITE URINE TEST

Quantofix sulfite test strips are available on Amazon.com and are designed to test sulfite levels in liquids such as urine, wine, beer, etc. Be cautious when ordering that you are in fact purchasing sulf-"ite" strips and not sulf-"ate" strips, they sound alike and can be confused for one another. Test your urine midstream 3 times daily and record your results, first making sure the pH of the urine is greater than 6.0 (you may need to use pH test strips to confirm). If the test strip shows any evidence of sulfites in your urine, this indicates that you need molybdenum supplementation.

For an adult, I recommend molybdenum supplementation from Thorne, Molybdenum Glycinate. Standard dosing in our office is 1 capsule 2 times per day with meals for 60 days, and then reduce the dose to 1 capsule per day ongoing for support. Once you have been on molybdenum support for 3 to 4 months, it is fine to stop taking the supplement and check your sulfite levels occasionally to monitor molybdenum levels. If molybdenum levels remain undetectable in your urine, you do not need additional molybdenum support. If sulfite levels return after a period of time, it simply indicates the need for continued molybdenum supplementation.

APPENDIX C:

———

SUPPLEMENT ORDERING INSTRUCTIONS

We use nutritional supplements every day in our practice. Because there are so many supplement companies from which to choose, it can get very confusing as to which product to use. As with any industry, the advertising and marketing slogans makes it difficult to separate the really good companies from the average ones. The companies listed here have passed our test; we use these exact products in our office every day with often miraculous results.

I have listed for you each company that I referenced in the protocols throughout this book. In a perfect world, I would have large warehouses all over the country and ship these from one location. With that said, we do offer our patients access to all the products we use in our office. The one hurdle is that patients must purchase products separately from each company versus having them sold from one website or store (unless you visit us in person).

The information that follows is intended to give you access to the top tier of nutritional supplements, so you can have the best chance of optimizing your genes and changing your life.

ELIXINOL HEMP CBD OIL

Elixinol Hemp Oil is the brand of CBD we have used with great success in our practice. Simply navigate to http://www.elixinol.com/ to purchase this product and it will be shipped directly to your front door.

NUTRIDYN

Nutridyn offers state-of-the-art, pharmaceutical grade supplements that helps address today's complex health challenges. Nutridyn batch tests every single raw ingredient – they test every batch, every time, before it is processed into a supplement. I'm not aware of any other company that puts that kind of expense and effort into product quality. Nutridyn products may be ordered by visiting the website https://www.Nutridyn.com/. You will need to register under our account number: **703900**.

ORGANO GOLD

Organo Gold products, including the black coffee I recommend for performing coffee enemas may be purchased at the following website: http://redmountain.organogold.com/beverages/.

APPENDIX D:

———

DIET GUIDELINES AND INSTRUCTIONS

ANTI-CANDIDA DIETARY GUIDELINES

FOODS TO AVOID

Additives, preservatives, artificial colorings and flavorings: Avoid consuming chemical preservatives and additives that are tough to pronounce. These are typically found in processed foods such as canned foods, frozen foods, prepared foods, and fast foods.

Alcohol: Alcohol is high in sugars that feed the yeast, so wine, beer, and spirits should all be avoided.

Caffeine: Caffeine gives the yeast a "boost" just as it does for you! Avoid caffeinated beverages and foods (including soda drinks, coffee, non-herbal teas, energy drinks, chocolate, etc.). Many of these products contain sugar and/or other sweeteners, which are not advisable when trying to rid the body of yeast.

Dairy: Aged cheeses are the worst culprits, although all dairy products should be avoided when trying to eliminate yeast. Avoid all margarine, milk products, and cheeses. Butter, ghee, and whey protein can be used in limited amounts (see "Foods to Eat in Moderation" for details).

Fermented and cultured foods: Avoid all fermented foods, including miso, tempeh, tamari/shoyu, sauerkraut, kimchee, coconut aminos, and Braggs Liquid Aminos. (These healthy foods can be introduced back into the diet when the gut is in a more balanced state.)

Fruits and fruit juices: Dried fruits should be completely avoided, because the sugars become more concentrated when the water content is removed. Avoid eating melons, strawberries, and grapes, which are very susceptible to molds. Canned and candied fruits are also not recommended, as they often contain added sugars, syrups, dyes, and preservatives. Avoid all fruit juices, including coconut water.

Gluten-containing foods and grains: Many people are sensitive or intolerant to gluten, without being aware of it. Consuming gluten-containing grains diverts the body's resources from combating an overgrowth of *Candida* because it is busy trying to manage the gluten overload. The main gluten-containing grains are wheat, barley, and rye, although spelt, kamut, amaranth, millet, and oats also tend to contain some levels of gluten. Avoid all wheat products, white bread, bleached flour products, and white rice.

Mushrooms: Mushrooms are a type of fungi. *Candida albicans* loves to feed on molds and fungi, which is why all mushroom products should be avoided during initial stages of treatment.

Non-organic animal products and eggs: These often contain steroids, pesticides, and hormones that disrupt the normal gut flora.

Nuts: Some nuts (especially peanuts and pistachios) are high in mold content. Nuts that were cracked a long time ago (e.g., bulk food products or prepackaged nuts) are also more susceptible to developing mold, which is particularly detrimental when *Candida albicans* is abundant in the body. Avoid all roasted and salted nuts, and peanuts and pistachios.

Spices and seasonings: Some spices can destroy the healthy bacteria in the gut, providing an environment for *Candida* to flourish. For this reason, pungent spices such as curry and hot peppers should be eliminated during initial stages of *Candida* treatment.

Sugars and sweets: Sugar feeds the yeast, therefore all products containing sugars (whether refined or natural sugars) should be avoided. This includes glucose, fructose, sucrose, high fructose corn syrup, etc. Avoid all refined sugar and candies.

Vinegar: Both white and apple cider vinegar should be eliminated because they are made in a yeast culture. All pickled products, commercial salad dressings, and other vinegar-containing foods should be removed from the diet.

FOODS TO EAT IN MODERATION

Dairy: Organic/grass-fed butter is okay every few days. Organic ghee can be used daily. High quality (low heat) pure whey protein is fine for those who tolerate it well.

Eggs: Limit to 2 organic or pasture-raised eggs per day. Best way for cooking is poached, hard-boiled, or soft-boiled.

Fruits: Limit fruit consumption, especially tropical fruits (mango, pineapple, papaya, etc.) which are high in natural sugars. If you continue to consume fruit, choose organic/unsprayed fruits. The best choices are green apples, pears, berries, pomegranates, avocados, lemons, and limes. You may also have apricots, cherries, guava, nectarines, papaya, peaches, plums, pineapple, and tangerines on occasion. Limit to 1 serving of fruit per day during initial treatment.

Non-gluten grains: Brown or wild rice is preferred as a substitute for wheat, rye, and barley-containing products. Quinoa and buckwheat are also good alternatives to gluten-containing breads, cereals, and pasta. Limit to 1 serving daily. If you eat gluten-free bread, limit to a maximum of 2 slices daily. Potatoes, corn, and tapioca flours are gluten-free; however, these foods are fairly starchy and should be limited or they may feed the yeast. Keep these limited to 1 serving only every few days. You may have organic sprouted corn tortillas or brown rice tortillas every few days. Also, almond flour, coconut flour, and quinoa flour are allowed as a substitute for gluten-containing grains/flours.

<u>Nuts and seeds</u>: Although some nuts and seeds should be avoided because of their high mold content, these foods are generally high in protein, which starves the yeast. It is best to crack and remove the shells from the nuts and seeds just before you intend to eat them, as this helps to preserve freshness and avoid molds. Alternatively, soaking them in water or spraying them with grapefruit seed extract or veggie wash may help to minimize the mold content. Eat only nuts and seeds that are raw, soaked, and/or sprouted. Examples are almonds, pecans, cashews, Brazil nuts, walnuts, sunflower seeds, pumpkin seeds, and chia seeds.

<u>Sweets and sweeteners</u>: Unpasteurized honey, raw coconut sugar, organic pure maple syrup, and unsulfured black-strap molasses may be used VERY OCCASIONALLY.

These vegetables should be limited to smaller portions:

- Corn
- Carrots
- Beets
- Peas
- Sweet potatoes
- Potatoes
- Yams
- Parsnips

FOODS TO EMPHASIZE

<u>Beverages</u>: Mineral water, herbal teas, green teas, white tea, dandelion tea, and fresh vegetable juices (from green leafy vegetables only).

<u>Oils</u>: High quality organic cold-pressed oils, preferably olive or coconut oil. The best oils for cooking are coconut oil or organic ghee. Flaxseed oil and olive oil are used unheated (great for salads or added to

already cooked foods).

Proteins: A diet rich in lean proteins helps to starve the yeast and restrict its growth, while providing essential nutrients and a sense of fullness. Organic animal sources of protein are recommended since non-organic products contain hormones and pesticides that create an extra toxic burden to the body. Processing these toxins diverts resources from combating yeast overgrowth. Emphasize organic/pasture-raised chicken, turkey, lamb, beef, wild game, and smaller sized low-mercury–containing fish.

Spices and seasonings: Chives, garlic, onion, parsley, laurel, marjoram, sage, thyme, savory, cumin, oregano, sea salt, kelp salt, and fresh herbs.

Sweetener: If a sweetener is desired, stevia can be used frequently.

Vegetables: Except for those listed earlier, vegetables should be eaten abundantly. Eat a wide variety to provide a balance of nutrients. Vegetables generally starve *Candida* of sugar and help to remove toxic yeast byproducts from the body. Those that are especially good at inhibiting *Candida* include garlic, onions, cabbage, broccoli, Brussel's sprouts, and kale. Other great vegetables to include are artichoke, asparagus, cauliflower, celery, chives, eggplant, endive, green pepper, leeks, radishes, spinach, zucchini, and tomatoes. Starchy vegetables, such as potatoes, sweet potatoes, yams, and other roots should be eliminated during initial stages of treatment, as they tend to have high sugar content that feeds yeast.

FOOD PROPORTIONS

40% Vegetables – As a rule of thumb, the vegetables on your plate for lunch and dinner should cover about half of your plate. This can be in the form of stews, salads, and steamed or sautéed vegetables.

40% Healthy Protein – This includes organic animal meats, fish, and eggs. If you are a vegetarian, your protein will come from beans, nuts, seeds, gluten-free grains like quinoa, plant-based protein powders (rice, pea, hemp-seed), and/or high quality whey protein powders if you tolerate them.

<u>10% Carbohydrates (root vegetables, legumes, beans, grains)</u> – A rule of thumb is no more than 3 servings per day (½ cup each serving) of these types of foods.

<u>10% Nuts, Seeds, and Fruit</u> – Limit fruits to 1 serving daily. Nuts/seeds should be limited to about ¼ cup daily.

Note: Always include plenty of healthy fats such as organic coconut oil, olive oil, and organic ghee.

COFFEE ENEMA INSTRUCTIONS

Talking about coffee enemas is a sure way to make people feel uncomfortable. "You want me to put coffee *where!?*" is the typical response. However, once we get past the unsavory thought of putting perfectly good coffee into our rectum, we can start to realize how useful these enemas can be. Whenever I need to help patients detoxify more effectively, coffee enemas are at the top of my list. The reason coffee enemas are effective is that when we retain coffee in the rectum for 5 to 10 minutes, the coffee goes directly to the liver via the portal vein, and once there, it triggers a powerful detoxification reaction. By performing coffee enemas, we not only rinse out the contents of the large intestine, which is cleansing in and of itself, but we also increase liver detoxification. This is an excellent tool for anyone who gets negative reactions when they try to detox or clean up their gut. Coffee enemas are also essential for anyone dealing with cancer.

For the equipment needed to perform coffee enemas, the list is pretty short. You need filtered water, coffee, and an enema kit. You can find enema kits at your local pharmacy, but there are better options online. The kit we recommend to our patients can be purchased online at the following web store: http://www.healthandyoga.com/html/product/enemaequipment.aspx. This kit is nice because it is easy to clean, is made from stainless steel, and the hose is a large diameter, medical-grade silicon. Other kits will do but this is the best. You can find the Organo Gold® coffee we recommend back in appendix C.

PREPARING A COFFEE ENEMA:

1. Put 1 quart of filtered water in a pan and carefully warm it up to body temperature. Water should be filtered, purified, reverse osmosis, etc. Tap water is not ideal because it contains plenty of toxins itself. Water that is warmer than your body temp will be uncomfortable and potentially seriously painful. Better to have water a little cooler than warmer than body temperature.

2. Open and mix into your pan two sachets of Organo Gold Gourmet Black Ganoderma Coffee.

3. (Optional) Add one tablespoon of unsulfured molasses since it helps in retaining the enemas and also increases the efficiency of detoxification.

PERFORMING A COFFEE ENEMA:

Next, carry your pan or pot and the enema kit into the bathroom and lay an old towel on the floor or bathtub. You may also want to bring a pillow and/or something to read.

Carefully pour the coffee from the pan into the measuring cup. Put your enema container in the sink with the catheter clamped closed.

Transfer the coffee from the pot/pan into the enema container. Loosen the clamp to allow the coffee to run out to the end of the catheter tip and re-clamp the bucket when all the air has been removed from the enema tubing.

Set the container on the counter or close the toilet lid and place it there. If you place the enema kit too high, there is excessive force of the enema and it can be very uncomfortable. I prefer putting the enema kit on the toilet seat because it causes less discomfort. Your results may vary.

Lie down on the floor/tub and gently insert the catheter. Always avoid petroleum products like KY or Vaseline, etc. If you need lubrication, either food-grade coconut, olive, or avocado oil will work fine. Gently insert the tube into the rectum a few inches and then release the clamp and let the first ½ of the quart (2 cups maximum) of the coffee flow in.

Clamp the tubing off as soon as there is the slightest amount of discomfort or fullness. Some prefer to roll to the right side and then to the left side a couple times, staying a few minutes on each side. Then lie flat and gently massage the abdomen.

Try to retain the enema for 10 minutes. Sometimes there will be an immediate urgency to get rid of it and that is fine. It helps to clean the stool out of the colon so that the next time around you can hold more of the enema. Never force yourself to retain it if you feel that you can't.

After you have clamped the tubing, remove the catheter tip and void when you have to. If you can hold it 10 minutes each time, fine. After you have emptied the bowel, proceed with the remaining ½ quart and likewise hold that for 10 minutes, if able, and then void.

The goal is to have two enemas, not exceeding ½ a quart (2 cups) each, that you are able to hold for 10 minutes each. After expelling the first enema, repeat another ½ quart enema, holding for another 10 minutes. One session consists of two ½ quart enemas, each held for 10 minutes. Your goal is to hold the enema for 10 minutes each time, but don't get discouraged if you are unable. 5 minutes of enema retention is still better than none.

At first, you may feel slightly jittery, although most patients find the enemas relaxing. Usually, the jitteriness lessens after about the third enema. If the jitteriness continues, this means you are making the coffee too strong. If you feel "wired" or hyper, or have palpitations or irregular heartbeats after a coffee enema, you should reduce the amount of coffee, usually by half for a few days or weeks. If you never experience the feeling of a squirting out up under the right ribs, and you can hold ½ of the quart enema easily for 10 minutes, you may need a slightly stronger solution of coffee or larger volume.

If a person is unable to get on the floor, the enema can be done in bed (with a bedpan and plenty of waterproof pads for easy clean-up). Or, it may be done as the person is semi-squatting or seated on the toilet. Merely insert the tube while seated and attempt to retain 10 minutes for two times per session as above. In this natural position of elimination, however, it is usually more difficult to retain it for 10 minutes.

Always discontinue the enemas if there is any adverse reaction whatsoever, and discuss it with your doctor.

LOW OXALATE DIET INFORMATION

To get the most up-to-date information on oxalate levels in foods, the Trying Low Oxalate Facebook group is your best bet. This group is run by Susan Owens, who is your best source for all oxalate-related research and info. Any Internet search you perform will give you some useful information. The following is an incomplete list of other websites that have useful information for those seeking to understand which foods contain high levels of oxalates:

http://www.lowoxalate.info/

https://kidneystones.uchicago.edu/how-to-eat-a-low-oxalate-diet/

http://whfoods.org/genpage.php?tname=george&dbid=48

HCL CHALLENGE

When using supplemental hydrochloric acid (HCl Support) for the first few times, please be sure to follow these directions carefully.

Always take HCl Support immediately after the meal when your normal digestive processes have started.

Day 1: Take one HCl Support tablet at the end of each meal all day long.

Day 2: Take two tablets at the end of each meal all day long.

Day 3 - Day 7: Continue increasing by one tablet per day, at the end of each meal, until you feel warmth in your stomach, or until you reach seven tablets per meal. Do not take more than seven tablets per meal.

When you experience the warming sensation in your stomach, reduce your dosage by one tablet.

NOTE: Drink 8 ounces of water with one tablespoon of baking soda if warming is uncomfortable.

IMPORTANT: This test should not be undertaken for those with gastritis or any recent history of gastric ulceration (stomach ulcers).

SIBO DIET INFORMATION

The best resource for an appropriate SIBO diet is the FODMAP/SCD diet guide created by Dr. Allison Siebecker. Her website, http://www.siboinfo.com is packed with useful information. You can find a free copy of her FODMAP/SCD diet on her website in the "Diet" section under the "Treatment" tab.

APPENDIX E:

FINDING A KINESIOLOGIST CHIROPRACTOR IN YOUR AREA

Visit the website http://www.icakusa.com/find-a-doctor and search for a doctor in your area. A kinesiologist chiropractor can be an enormous asset for you in your quest to regain your health. I am a kinesiologist chiropractor and it allows me to help people in miraculous ways. Applied kinesiology practitioners have special training to help you in ways other doctors simply cannot. I often recommend our patients find a doctor in their area to assist with treating their hiatal hernia and helping with their ICV. As discussed in earlier chapters, these two aspects of our health are critical for optimum digestion, and yet they are often completely overlooked. If you want the best health you can imagine, you need to branch out and meet people in your area who are skilled and who can assist you directly. Either come see us in Boise, or find a doctor near you who can use applied kinesiology to give your health that needed boost.

www.ingramcontent.com/pod-product-compliance
Lightning Source LLC
Chambersburg PA
CBHW060031030426
42334CB00019B/2281